Food and Drink in Archaeology 4
University of Exeter Postgraduate Conference 2010

Food and Drink in Archaeology 4

University of Exeter Postgraduate Conference 2010

Edited by
Wendy Howard, Kirsten Bedigan and Ben Jervis

Prospect Books
2015

First published in Great Britain in 2015 by Prospect Books, 26 Parke Road, London SW13 9NG.

© 2015 as a collection Prospect Books.
© 2015 in individual articles rests with the authors.

The authors assert their moral right to be identified as authors in accordance with the Copyright, Designs & Patents Act 1988. No part of this publication may be reproduced, stored in a retrieval system or transmitted in any form or by any means, electronic, mechanical, photocopying, recording or otherwise, without the prior permission of the copyright holders.

ISBN 978-1-909248-35-9

The illustration on the cover is of a harvest jug from north Devon, 1702. It is copyright of the Royal Albert Memorial Museum and Art Gallery and Exeter City Council.

For more information about Prospect Books: https://prospectbooks.co.uk.

Printed in the United Kingdom by Jellyfish Solutions Ltd.

Contents

List of Figures — 7

List of Tables — 9

Ertebølle Cuisine: A Freshwater Radiocarbon Reservoir Effect in Mesolithic Food Crusts from Northern Germany
Bente Philippsen and Jan Heinemeier — 13

Fun and Feasting: Contextualizing the Animal Remains from the Kabeirion at Thebes
Kirsten Bedigan — 30

Splitting Hares! Investigating Anthropogenic Modification Signatures on Leporid Bones, using Actualistic Experiments to Improve Identifying Small Mammal Exploitation by Humans
Wendy Howard — 40

Honey Hunting, Beekeeping and the Uses and Role of Bee Products in British Prehistory
Magnhild Peggy Gilje — 56

The Craft of the Maltster
Merryn Dineley — 63

Pottery as Evidence for Lifestyles in Early Iron Age Corinthia (*c.* 1100–690 BC): Water, Commensality and Ownership
Sam Farnham — 72

The Preliminary Results from a Herculaneum Sewer: What's Inside? Why? And what Can it Tell us about Roman Diet?
Erica Rowan — 81

The 1270 Durrës Earthquake Victims in the Roman Amphitheatre Excavations: a Global Palaeonutritional Study of an Anthropological and Archaeological Sample
Sara Santoro, Antonietta Buglione, Giovanni De Venuto, Paola Iacumin, Barbara Sassi and Loretana Salvadei — 95

Provisioning and Diet in Hamwic (Mid-Saxon Southampton): New Data and New Perspectives
Ben Jervis   110

Provisioning Shakespeare's Audiences: Food and Drink in the London Playhouses of the Sixteenth and Seventeenth Centuries
Julian Bowsher   128

Shorter Contributions

Agriculture in Prehistoric Croatia and Serbia: Continuity and Change
Kelly Reed   139

The Processing and Treatment of Drinking Water in Iberia (*c.* Sixth–Second Centuries BC)
Meritxell Oliach Fàbregas   143

Food Processing and Consumption Spaces: the Case of Molí d'Espígol (Catalonia, Spain) in the Third Century BC
Meritxell Monrós and Pilar Camañes   149

Eating and Drinking with the Dead: Archaeological Evidence for Commemorative Rites at the Cemeteries of Tarraco (Tarragona, Spain) from the First to the Fourth Centuries AD
Judit Ciurana Prast   154

Relating Meat and Fish Consumption to Climate Change on the Swahili Coast (AD 700–1500)
Eréndira Quintana Morales   158

'Reare the Goose': Recognizing a Standard Method of Carcase Dismemberment
Louisa Gidney   164

List of Figures

1.1	Stable isotope values of experimental and archaeological food crusts	18
1.2	Radiocarbon dating of archaeological samples from Schlamersdorf	22
1.3	Radiocarbon dating of archaeological samples from Kayhude	23
2.1	Chronological distribution for cattle, sheep/goats and red deer at the Kabeirion	31
2.2	Chronological distribution for cattle, sheep/goat and deer (red, fallow and roe) knucklebones at the Kabeirion	33
3.1	Cooking the rabbits by spit-roasting, suspending them above a pre-heated fire and by pit-roasting	43
3.2	Area chipped off the anconeus during linear hyperextension of the left elbow	46
3.3	a) Burning discoloration on a distal tibia; b) Crazing on the humeral head of a pit-roasted rabbit; c and d) Breaks at the spine/body junction of spit-roasted rabbit scapulae, attributed to forelimb disarticulation	50
3.4	The relative frequency of damage to the proximal ulnae of leporids from two control assemblages and from two archaeological sites	51
5.1	Sections through barley grain	64
5.2	Turning the malt at Bury Maltings with a duck foot rake	67
5.3	Scanning electric microscope image of a carbonised grain, with missing embryo visible on the right, from Balbridie, Fife, Scotland	69
6.1	Pottery deposited in burial contexts classified by function as percentages, 875–690 BC	74
6.2	Pottery deposited in sanctuary contexts classified by function as percentages, 900–690 BC	76
6.3	Topographical map of the natural water sources in Corinth and the 8th- and 7th-century wells with some post EIA structures	77
7.1	Insula Orientalis II and the Cardo V sewer (Sosandra/HCP)	82
7.2	Ancient corneous wedge clams (*Donacilla cornea*) from quadrant 13–14	91
7.3	Ancient olive stone fragments from quadrant 3–4	91
8.1	The Roman amphitheatre in Dürrres. To the north-east is a necropolis, to the south a glass kiln and to the east a medieval building	97
8.2	Map of archaeological features in the southern part of the Dürres amphitheatre (area B)	98
8.3	Nitrogen and carbon isotope composition of collagen.	103
8.4	The medieval animal bone samples according NISP and MNI	105
8.5	The survival curve for sheep/goat	105
8.6	The anatomical distribution for cattle, pig and sheep/goats	106

9.1	a) The location of Hamwic within Southampton; b) Typical ceramic vessels from Hamwic	111
9.2	Distribution of phase 2 wares within Hamwic	114
9.3	Ceramic use patterns in Hamwic	120
9.4	a) Temporal trends in sooting type in Hamwic; b) Temporal trends in the pottery function in Hamwic	123
10.1	Map of London	129
11.1	Site locations within Croatia and Serbia	139
12.1	Cistern at Tossal de les Tenalles (Sidamón)	144
12.2	Filtration system documented at Puig Castellet (Lloret de Mar)	145
12.3	Puig de Sant Andreu, detail of step used for cleaning the cistern	146
13.1	Geographical location and the general plan of Molí d'Espígol	150
13.2	Singular Building C plan and graphics quantifying materials found	151
13.3	Singular Building A plan and graphics showing the materials found	152
14.1	Archaeological plan of the Roman city of Tarraco	155
14.2	Reenactment of a *silicernium* by the Cultural Association of Saint Fructuosus	155
15.1	The ratio of the total number of fish bones to domesticated animal bones over time in three Swahili sites	159
15.2	Conductivity levels through time, inferred from the diatom record	160
15.3	Trends in the ratio of fish bone to domesticated animal bone and the mean trophic level of fish bone throughout the occupation at Shanga	162
16.1	Two fragments of archaeological goose sternum from Richmond, showing the characteristic slice through the bone parallel to the spine	165
16.2	View of the same goose sternum (from Richmond) showing the broken spine	166
16.3	Modern goose sterna: three carved by the 'reare the goose' method and one by the modern method	167

List of Tables

1.1	Food crust experiments with mixed ingredients	14
1.2	^{14}C and stable isotope measurements of modern samples	19
1.3	Radiocarbon dating and stable isotope measurements of archaeological samples from Kayhude LA 8 and Schlamersdorf LA 5	20
1.4	Examples of hunter-gatherer pottery in northern Europe	25
2.1	Estimated gender and age categories for all species excavated at the sanctuary	32
2.2	Fabric, species and processing information for the knucklebones based upon the archaeological and epigraphic evidence	35
2.3	Approximate totals for the metal and terracotta animal figurines from the sanctuary	36
3.1	Uncooked, fleshed rabbit, subjected to linear hyperextension	45
3.2	Uncooked, fleshed rabbit, subjected to twisting disarticulation	45
3.3	Spit-roasted rabbit, subjected to linear hyperextension	47
3.4	Spit-roasted rabbit, subjected to twisting disarticulation	47
3.5	Pit-roasted rabbit, subjected to linear hyperextension	48
3.6	Pit-roasted rabbit, subjected to disarticulation by twisting	48
6.1	Absolute and relative dates of the periods mentioned in the text	72
7.1	Mineralized material	86
7.2	Carbonized material	87
7.3	Waterlogged material	88
7.4	Seashell material	88
8.1	Gender and age list of earthquake victims	100
8.2	Isotopic ratios (‰) of carbon and oxygen in the carbonate apatite, isotope composition of carbon and nitrogen in the collagen and C/N ratio	103
9.1	Hamwic ceramic phases	113
9.2	The composition of phase 2 pottery assemblages at sites in Hamwic	116
9.3	The spread of phase 2 wares through Hamwic	117
9.4	Pottery use in phase 1	118
9.5	Sandy ware use (phase 2)	119
9.6	Chalk tempered ware use (phase 2)	119
9.7	Phase 3 vessel use	120
9.8	Imported vessel use	122
9.9	Results of residue analysis	124
11.1	Relative abundance of crop remains recovered from 18 sites within Croatia and Serbia	140

Preface

These proceedings derive from the Fourth Food and Drink in Archaeology Postgraduate Conference, which was held at the University of Exeter on 23 April 2010. As conferences go, it had the unusual, perhaps unique, distinction for Devon (or indeed anywhere in the United Kingdom) in that it was disrupted by the eruption of the Eyjafjallajökull volcano in Iceland. The impact of its ash cloud on flights prevented a number of European delegates from countries such as Italy, Spain, Scandinavia, and even Scotland, from attending the conference, with the subsequent loss of several papers, and the conference organisers are grateful to those who presented papers at the conference (some at the last minute on behalf of the orginal authors) or who still managed to attend despite these setbacks.

The papers in this volume are representative of the impressive diversity of subjects presented at the conference. Chronologically, they comprise papers that address aspects of food and drink from early prehistory, through later prehistory to the historic period and the Romans, as well as medieval and modern times, while geographically deriving from a diverse range of locations that cover several continents. Consequently, this volume has been arranged chronologically, firstly for the full-length papers, and then likewise for the shorter contributions; these latter based on posters presented at the conference. The topics addressed include both direct and indirect evidence for food- and drink-related issues in the past. Between them, these papers examine the dietary choices people made, or were restricted to, how they processed, prepared, cooked and consumed such items, and the contexts in which they were undertaken. The diverse approaches employed range from scientific techniques, multifaceted studies, ethnographic analogy and experimental archaeology, and encompass techniques specific to examining the ceramic material culture, human and faunal osteological data, botanical and palaeoenvironmental evidence. The result is a volume that substantially contributes to further our understanding of food and drink in archaeology.

Finally, thanks must go to those who helped with the conference and made it a success on the day, and to all those who presented papers and posters or attended. Many thanks also to all those anonymous experts who kindly peer reviewed these papers, to publisher Tom Jaine for his enthusiasm and patience, and to Naomi Sykes for her advice and guidance with this publication.

Wendy Howard,
University of Exeter

Ertebølle Cuisine: A Freshwater Radiocarbon Reservoir Effect in Mesolithic Food Crusts from Northern Germany

Bente Philippsen and Jan Heinemeier
AMS ^{14}C Dating Centre, Department of Physics and Astronomy, University of Aarhus

Pottery is one of the most important materials for prehistoric archaeology and is often used to define cultures and to study cultural contacts and developments. It was also a remarkable innovation for Terminal Mesolithic 'cuisine': boiling in vessels over direct heat made food resources available that could not otherwise be digested, whilst preserving all nutrients in liquid foodstuffs. For reliable ^{14}C dating of food crusts on pottery, reservoir effects have to be ruled out or quantified. It is thus important to find out whether the food crust contains components of marine or freshwater resources. The food crusts analysed in this study are from pottery found in Schleswig-Holstein (northern Germany), belonging to the Terminal Mesolithic Ertebølle Culture. This hunter-gatherer culture was the first culture in northern Germany, Poland and southern Scandinavia that adopted pottery production.

^{14}C dating of food remains in pottery from two inland sites resulted in ages more than 500 years older than those from coastal settlements (Hartz 1996; Clausen 2008). Because of this a reservoir effect was suspected (Hartz and Lübke 2006). The two sites are Schlamersdorf LA 5 on the river Trave and Kayhude LA 8 on the river Alster (Hartz 1997; Clausen 2008); both rivers are characterized by hard water. Remains of fish and fishing gear had been excavated at these sites and the consumption of freshwater fish is typical for the Late Mesolithic, so it is probable that freshwater fish was cooked in the pots.

Modern samples (water, plants and animals) from both rivers were collected in 2007–2009 and ^{14}C dated to determine whether a reservoir effect in that area is likely, and of what magnitude it could be. Food crusts from different ingredients and mixtures of ingredients were analysed to find the relation between the isotopic values of the ingredients and of the food crust (Table 1.1). The reservoir ages of ingredients and food crusts were compared as well. In order to quantify the effect on ancient material, archaeological samples of terrestrial and freshwater origin as well as archaeological food crusts have been ^{14}C dated.

Table 1.1. Food crust experiments with mixed ingredients. For each stew, the ingredients are listed. $\delta^{13}C$ and $\delta^{15}N$ values are given for the uncooked ingredients. From the relative amounts of the ingredients and their respective carbon and nitrogen content, an expected value for the homogeneous mixture was calculated. Different samples of the food and food crusts were taken. 'Crust' denotes a random sample from the inside of the pot; which ingredients were unidentifiable – just what you would find on an archaeological potsherd. Two other food crusts were made of only one ingredient each: freshwater fish (roach) and wild boar meat. The results for these two are given in Table 1.2.

Pot	Ingredient / Material	Mass [g]	Percentage of solids	$\delta^{13}C$ VPDB (‰)	$\delta^{15}N$ AIR (‰)
1	Celery stalks	128	37.9	-28.82	10.45
	Carrots	90	26.6	-26.89	3.63
	Brussels sprouts	120	35.5	-29.04	8.07
	Water	119	—		
	Expected			-28.04	7.95
	Cooked mixture			-27.63	7.88
	Crust			-28.53	10.09
	Cooked Brussels sprouts			-27.88	9.12
	Charred Brussels sprouts			-27.23	9.77
	Cooked carrot			-27.59	4.73
	Charred carrot			-27.53	5.19
2	Celery	157	49.7	-28.82	10.45
	Cod	159	50.3	-18.73	15.15
	Water	405	—		
	Expected			-22.92	14.91
	Cooked celery			-28.2	15.84
	Cooked cod			-18.99	15.29
	Cooked mixture			-19.61	14.97
	Crust 1			-21.63	15.86
	Crust 2			-19.08	16.53
	Crust 3			-20.34	12.45
	Crust 4			-18.57	17.44
	Crust (boiled over)			-25.14	12.87
	Outer crust			-23.38	12.36
3	Rocket	65	30.2	-30.27	9.02
	Chard	60	27.9	-30.17	2.05
	Fish (Roach)	90	41.9	-22.3	14.86

Ertebølle Cuisine

Pot	Ingredient / Material	Mass [g]	Percentage of solids	δ¹³C VPDB (‰)	δ¹⁵N AIR (‰)
	Water	575	—		
	Expected			-27.11	13.13
	Cooked vegetables			-27.73	1.89
	Cooked fish			-21.55	13.62
	Fishbone (cooked)			-18.59	13.19
	Cooked mixture			-23.12	14.02
	Crust 1			-26.18	12.73
	Crust 2			-24.81	13.08
4	Roe deer meat	180	50	-26.24	8.69
	Rocket	90	25	-30.27	9.02
	Chard	90	25	-30.28	2.05
	Water	930	—		
	Expected			-29.32	9.4
	Cooked vegetables			-28.38	-1.9
	Cooked meat			-26.16	8.27
	Cooked mixture 1			-26.63	7.56
	Crust 1			-27.45	5.02
	Crust 2			-25.57	9.85
	Soot from outside			-25.16	9.56
5	Plaice	111	50	-18.53	14.03
	Roe deer meat	111	50	-26.24	8.69
	Water	850	—		
	Expected			-22.38	11.42
	Cooked fish			-18.61	13.96
	Cooked meat			-26.03	8.24
	Boiled over (froth)			-19.76	13.4
	Crust (with fish & meat)			-25.9	8.04
	Crust (upper rim)			-20.14	13.43
	Crust 1			-19.48	13.94
	Crust 2			-19.42	13.94
	Crust 3			-21.14	11.89

Ertebølle Cuisine

Radiocarbon dating and reservoir effects

A terrestrial sample's carbon derives from the atmosphere. When a sample obtains its carbon from a reservoir with a lower ^{14}C concentration than the atmosphere, ^{14}C ages that are too high will be obtained. The difference between the ^{14}C age of a sample from such a reservoir and the ^{14}C age of a contemporaneous terrestrial sample is called the reservoir age. A marine reservoir age of 400 years is common for Danish and northern German coastal areas, as well as for most of the North Atlantic region (Tauber 1979; Heier-Nielsen et al. 1995).

Another example of a reservoir effect is the hard water effect (Godwin 1951; Deevey et al. 1954). Hard water contains considerable amounts of ^{14}C dead carbon: dissolved carbonate from rocks and deposits in the underground has infinite ages on the ^{14}C time scale. The initial ^{14}C concentration of an organism living in hard water is thus lower than that of a terrestrial sample (Clark and Fritz 1997; Fontes and Garnier 1979). The hardwater effect can potentially lead to very high reservoir ages, both in samples of these organisms and for samples from humans who eat fish from hard water (Cook et al. 2001; Smits and van der Plicht 2009; Olsen et al. 2010). A hardwater effect in food crusts on pottery was first proposed by Fischer and Heinemeier (2003), and for example found by Boudin et al. (in press) to be 320±160 ^{14}C years for Swifterbant pottery from Belgium.

Stable isotope analysis

Both carbon and nitrogen have two naturally occurring stable isotopes: ^{12}C, ^{13}C and ^{14}N, ^{15}N. The mass difference between isotopes leads to different chemical reaction rates. 'Isotopic fractionation' is the enrichment or depletion of a certain isotope during a chemical reaction or physical or biological process. Stable isotope contents are expressed as rare/abundant ratios ($^{13}C/^{12}C$ and $^{15}N/^{14}N$), relative to this ratio for a standard, expressed as delta values ($\delta^{13}C$ and $\delta^{15}N$) in permil deviation, for example $\delta^{13}C = (^{13}R_{sam} - ^{13}R_{std}) / (^{13}R_{std}) * 1000‰$. The standards for ^{13}C and ^{15}N are VPDB and AIR, respectively (Craig 1957; Mariotti 1983).

^{13}C can be used to differentiate between marine and terrestrial food sources as the food chains in these environments begin with different $^{13}C/^{12}C$ ratios. Atmospheric CO_2 has $\delta^{13}C \approx -7‰$, marine CO_2 has $\delta^{13}C \approx 0‰$ because of fractionation in the CO_2 exchange across the air-water boundary. The type of photosynthesis (C3) that is used by water plants and most plants in temperate Europe leads to a fractionation of about -18‰. Terrestrial plants thus have $\delta^{13}C \approx -25‰$, marine plants $\approx -18‰$. There is a shift of about +5‰ from food source to consumer bone collagen. Humans who live mainly on marine food have $\delta^{13}C$ values in their bone collagen of about -13‰ (Lanting and van der Plicht 1995/6; Arneborg et al. 1999). A predominantly terrestrial diet leads to $\delta^{13}C \approx -21‰$ in bone collagen.

In the case of ^{15}N, there is enrichment of about 3‰ with each step in trophic level (Ambrose 2001). In aquatic systems, food chains are generally longer than in terrestrial systems, resulting in more ^{15}N enrichment steps. Humans who live on a 100% aquatic diet may have δ^{15}N = 16–18‰ in their bone collagen (Schoeninger et al. 1983; Cook et al. 2001).

Thus, the combination of δ^{13}C and δ^{15}N values could, in principle, be used to identify the ingredients of a food crust: δ^{13}C differentiates marine and terrestrial (including freshwater) systems, whereas δ^{15}N differentiates between water (including freshwater) and land. A combined measurement is thus needed to identify freshwater samples. The identification of a sample's origin can be used to correct a ^{14}C measurement for the reservoir effect (Arneborg et al. 1999; Cook et al. 2001). Obvious difficulties are, however, identifying individual food components in a mixture as well as fractionation in the charring of food crusts.

Methods

For the dating of water samples, dissolved inorganic carbon (DIC) was extracted as CO_2 and reduced to graphite for radiocarbon dating (Boaretto et al. 1998). Some water plants from the rivers have been analysed to simulate the first step in the food chain, and fish, shells and a crayfish have also been examined. Bulk samples were analysed, but in the case of fishbone only the collagen fraction was used.

It has been tested whether the ^{14}C age of a food crust is the same as that of the cooking ingredients. One could imagine that the process of cooking and scorching leads to effects that alter the ^{14}C age (for example, contamination), so both ingredients and food crusts have been ^{14}C dated. The stable isotope ratios δ^{13}C and δ^{15}N were also measured for these samples. The food crusts were produced in copies of Stone Age pottery made using prehistoric methods (see Philippsen (2010) for details).

From the archaeological sites, terrestrial samples, fishbones and food crusts were analysed. Food crusts, wood and charcoal samples were pre-treated with the method described in Olsson (1976). Collagen from bones and fishbones was extracted with a modified Longin-method and purified by ultrafiltration (Longin 1971; Brown et al. 1988; Jørkov et al. 2007; Kanstrup 2008). The pre-treated samples were combusted to CO_2. Part of it could be used for δ^{13}C measurements on a GV Instruments IsoPrime stable isotope mass spectrometer. A fraction corresponding to 1 mg carbon was converted to graphite by reduction with H_2 in the presence of a cobalt catalyst. A fraction of pre-treated bone and food crust samples was measured directly on the mass spectrometer, yielding both δ^{13}C and δ^{15}N.

AMS ^{14}C measurements were carried out using the EN tandem accelerator at Aarhus University. The dating results are reported according to international convention (Stuiver and Polach 1977) as conventional ^{14}C dates in ^{14}C yr BP (before AD 1950) based on the measured ^{14}C/^{13}C ratio corrected for the natural isotopic fractionation by normalizing the result to the standard δ^{13}C value of -25‰ PDB (Andersen et al. 1989). The radiocarbon determinations on archaeological material were calibrated with OxCal v4.1.4 (Bronk Ramsey 2009) using the terrestrial calibration curve IntCal09 (Reimer et al. 2009).

Results and discussion
Stable isotopes
Figure 1.1 shows the stable isotope results of the experimental and archaeological food crusts. In some cases, different samples from the same pot have very different stable isotope values. Several measured values differ a lot from the expected values that are calculated from the relative contributions of the ingredients to the carbon and nitrogen of the food crust. This is to be expected, given that food crusts likely derive from multiple cooking events and, therefore, that the analysed potsherd crust may not be representative of the meal prepared in the pot.

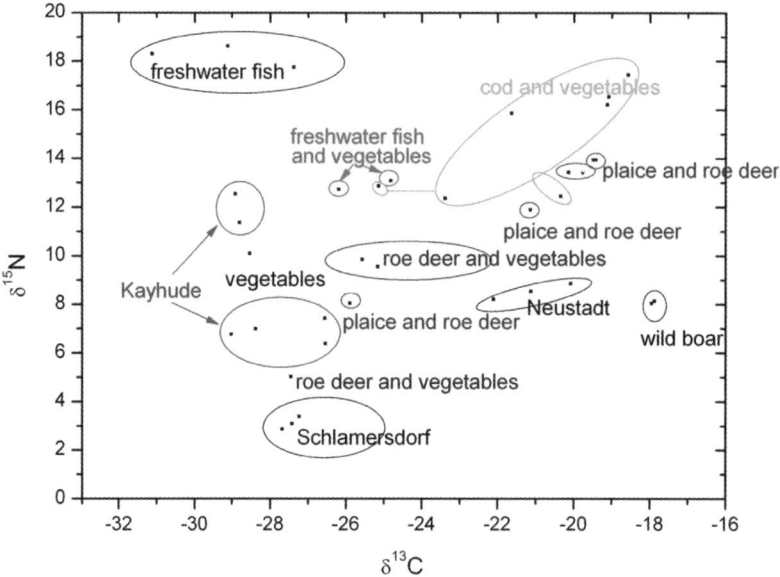

Figure 1.1. Stable isotope values of experimental and archaeological food crusts. The data of experimental food crusts are marked with the names of the ingredients. The data of archaeological food crusts are marked with the name of the site. Neustadt is a coastal site so that marine fish is one possible ingredient for this food crust.

The $\delta^{13}C$ value of the wild boar food crust is much less negative than expected. This wild boar was probably fed with maize, which is a C4 plant with very different $\delta^{13}C$ values (c. -13‰). The $\delta^{13}C$ values of the archaeological food crusts from Schlamersdorf and Kayhude are comparable to those found by Fischer and Heinemeier (2003) and Smits and van der Plicht (2009): they range between -29 and -27‰, indicating terrestrial to freshwater origin.

The $\delta^{15}N$ values span a range of 3 to 13‰. $\delta^{15}N$ values in archaeological food crusts, especially in those from Schlamersdorf, are lower than those in experimental food crusts. Maybe these values can be used for a characterization of the preservation status of a potsherd food crust. Further studies are needed to develop reliable criteria for this effect.

^{14}C dating
Modern samples

Table 1.2 shows the broad range of ^{14}C ages for modern samples. It is evident that there is no uniform reservoir age for the water, plants or animals from the same river. Recent terrestrial samples have negative ^{14}C ages, caused by the increase of atmospheric ^{14}C concentration due to nuclear bomb tests since the late 1950s (Fischer and Heinemeier 2003). The crust made of a roach, caught in 2007, with a ^{14}C age of 285 ± 30 BP, had a ^{14}C age of 330 ± 20 BP. Similarly, the wild boar food crust has no age offset, as expected for a modern terrestrial sample. We can thus conclude that ingredients and crust have the same reservoir age.

Table 1.2. ^{14}C and stable isotope measurements of modern samples. The water plants and animals were collected live in 2007 and 2008. °dH for the water samples denotes the carbonate hardness, estimated with an aquarium test kit and expressed in German degrees (1°dH =17.848 milligrams of calcium carbonate per litre of water). DIC is dissolved inorganic carbon from the water samples. $\delta^{13}C$ values marked with DI were measured on sample CO2, while those marked with EA were measured on the pre-treated samples.

Lab No. AAR-	River	Sample type	^{14}C Age (uncal. yr BP)	$\delta^{13}C$ (‰ wrt VPDB)	$\delta^{15}N$ (‰ wrt AIR)	Misc.
11780	Trave	Water DIC (Aug 07)	1170±60	-13.59 (DI)		7.5°dH
12882	Trave	Water DIC (Sep 08)	1990±40	-11.30 (DI)		7.5°dH
13611	Trave	Water DIC (Feb 09)	1175±30	-8.94 (DI)		8.0°dH
11779	Alster	Water DIC (Aug 07)	1965±30	-14.96 (DI)		5.0°dH
12881	Alster	Water DIC (Sep 08)	2620±50	-10.92 (DI)		4.5°dH
13612	Alster	Water DIC (Feb 09)	1520±35	-14.85 (DI)		5.0°dH
12870	Trave	Underwater plant	-75±35	-25.42 (EA)	9.22	
12871	Trave	Water plant	880±35	-28.67 (EA)	13.67	
12872	Trave	Underwater plant	1700±55	-17.65 (EA)	8.50	

Lab No. AAR-	River	Sample type	^{14}C Age (uncal. yr BP)	δ^{13}C (‰ wrt VPDB)	δ^{15}N (‰ wrt AIR)	Misc.
11394	Trave	Fishbone (Roach)	285±30	-26.00 (EA) -25.91 (DI)	15.02	
12875	Trave	Fish (Spined loach)	1665±40	-27.18 (EA)	17.88	
12876	Trave	Crayfish	1365±40	-23.65 (EA)	11.54	
12873	Alster	Underwater plant	2275±40	-31.48 (EA)	14.26	
11461	Alster	Snail-shell	435±30	-15.36 (DI)		
11462	Alster	Fishbone (roach)	225±30	-25.29 (EA) -25.46 (DI)	12.24	
11414	Trave	Fish food crust (roach)	330±20	-28.13 (EA) -30.47 (DI)	13.30	
11411	(Trave)	Wild boar food crust	-535±55	-17.88 (EA) -18.03 (DI)	8.13	

Table 1.3. Radiocarbon dating and stable isotope measurements of archaeological samples from Kayhude LA 8 and Schlamersdorf LA 5, Schleswig-Holstein, northern Germany. The 'humic fraction' is the alkali-soluble fraction of the food crust. This fraction is likely to be contaminated with humic substances from the soil. δ^{13}C values marked with DI were measured on sample CO2, while those marked with EA were measured on the pre-treated samples with the mass spectrometer in combination with an elemental analyser. From a red deer bone, two subsamples have been extracted and pre-treated individually to illustrate the variation in radiocarbon dates of the same sample.

Lab no. AAR-	Name and material	^{14}C age Yr BP	cal. age BC (95.4%)	δ^{13}C (‰ wrt VPDB)	δ^{15}N (‰ wrt AIR)
	Kayhude (Alster)				
11403	Food crust	5695±55	4690-4370	-28.38 (EA) -28.63 (DI)	6.99
11403	Food crust, humic fraction	6740±160	5980-5380		
11404	Food crust	6090±55	5210-4850	-28.90 (EA) -28.90 (DI)	12.54
11404	Food crust, humic fraction	6420±65	5610-5320		
11479	Food crust	5350±110	4440-3960	-26.53 (EA) -24.83 (DI)	6.38
11480	Charcoal	5435±40	4360-4180		
11695	Fishbone	8510±80	7730-7370	-22.41 (DI)	

Ertebølle Cuisine

Lab no. AAR-	Name and material	^{14}C age Yr BP	cal. age BC (95.4%)	$\delta^{13}C$ (‰ wrt VPDB)	$\delta^{15}N$ (‰ wrt AIR)
Schlamersdorf (Trave)					
11398	Wildcat	5685±60	4690-4370	-19.16 (EA) -19.27 (DI)	6.49
11399	Beaver	6480±90	5620-5300	-22.54 (EA) -22.42 (DI)	4.68
11400	Wild boar	6035±60	5200-4780	-21.20 (EA) -21.39 (DI)	5.01
11402	Wood	5640±50	4581-4350	-26.49 (DI)	
11405	Wood	5760±50	4720-4490	-27.25 (DI)	
11406	Wood	5820±45	4780-4550	-28.78 (DI)	
11407	Burnt wood	5750±90	4790-4370	-27.03 (DI)	
11408	Wood	5640±50	4580-4360	-27.47 (DI)	
11476	Red deer (a)	6275±65	5460-5050	-23.63 (DI)	
11476	Red deer (b)	6370±65	5470-5220	-23.54 (DI)	
11481	Food crust	6850±120	5990-5560	-27.23 (EA)	3.95
11481	Outer crust	5190±110	4320-3710	-28.01 (EA)	3.39
11482	Food crust	5590±110	4710-4240	-27.04 (EA)	2.86
11483	Food crust			-27.36 (EA) -27.62 (DI)	3.09
11483	Plant rest from sherd	5985±50	5000-4730		
11484	Food crust	5830±180	5210-4340	-27.46 (EA)	1.88
11842	Fishbone	7640±65	6630-6400	-26.78 (DI)	
11844	Fishbone	7620±110	6680-6240		

Archaeological samples

The terrestrial age range of Schlamersdorf (Figure 1.2) complies with earlier dates from this site, derived from charcoal (Hartz 1993). The broad range of terrestrial ages, probably caused by uncertainties in the stratigraphy, makes it difficult to calculate reservoir ages. It is obvious, though, that fishbones are significantly older than other samples. Three food crusts had previously been dated to around 5300 cal. BC (Hartz 1996); their $\delta^{13}C$ values between -28.6 and -31.9‰ indicate freshwater ingredients. Two of the three food crusts we radiocarbon-dated from that site are from 4000–5000 BC, and one was from 5600–6000 BC. An interesting case is the potsherd AAR–11481 where both inner and outer crusts have been dated. If one assumes that the outer crust is soot from the cooking fire, then it should give the date of cooking, or an older date in case old wood had been used. The reservoir effect would, in this case, be approximately 2000 years. As this outer crust is younger than all the other terrestrial samples, we will examine it more

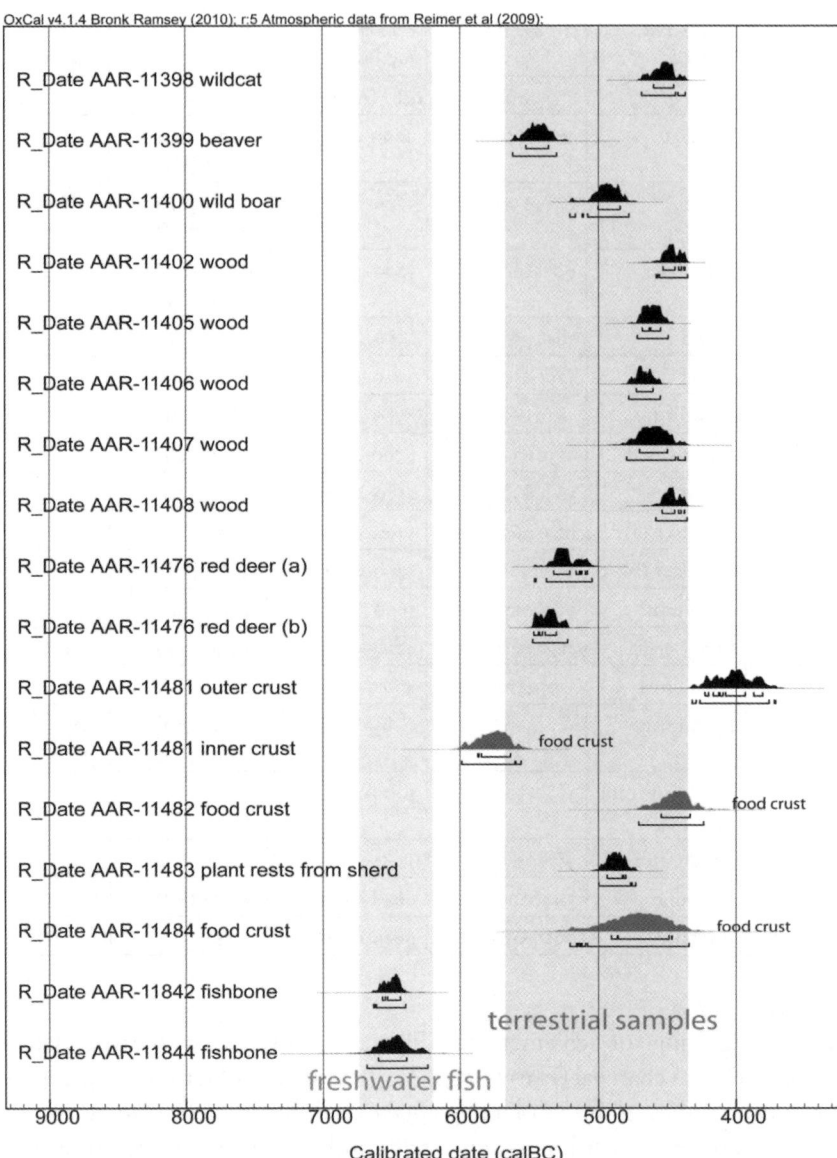

Figure 1.2. Radiocarbon dating of archaeological samples from Schlamersdorf. The age ranges of fresh-water and terrestrial samples are shaded and radiocarbon datings of food crusts on pottery are coloured red. There is a big variability of terrestrial ages, which might be caused by the unsure stratigraphy. The fishbones are significantly older than the terrestrial samples. The food crust dates are within the ages of terrestrial samples or slightly older. One striking example is the potsherd AAR-11481 where both inner and outer crusts have been dated. The large age difference between those makes a reservoir effect very likely.

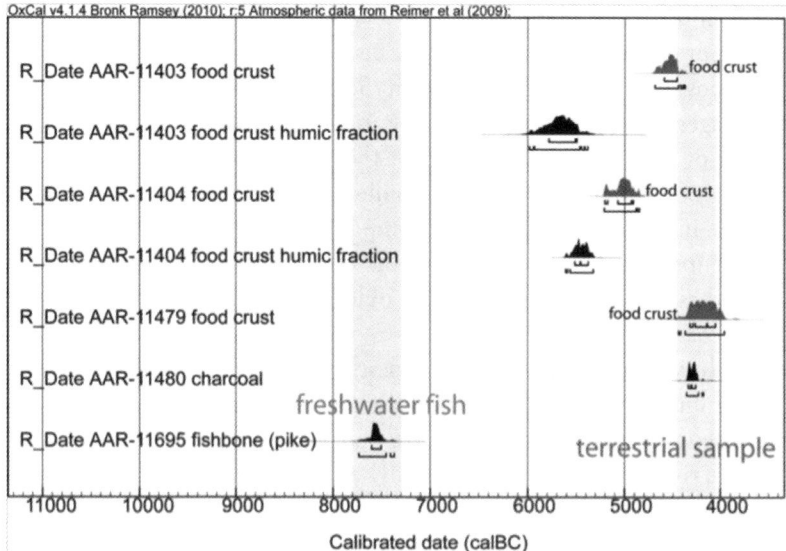

Figure 1.3. Radiocarbon dating of archaeological samples from Kayhude. The age ranges of fresh-water and terrestrial samples are shaded and radiocarbon datings of food crusts on pottery are coloured red. The samples were taken from a stone paving that seemed to be relatively undisturbed, so that it is likely here that all dated samples were contemporaneous. The fishbones are significantly older than the terrestrial samples. The food crusts have the same apparent age as the terrestrial sample or are older, though none of the food crusts is as old as the fishbone.

closely to find out if it really is soot, or just some more recent contamination. In one of the sherds, AAR–11483, we were lucky to find some plant remains that presumably had been incorporated in the clay during the forming of the pottery. Unfortunately, the food crust sample of AAR–11483 was lost during dating.

In Kayhude, the samples were collected from a relatively undisturbed stone paving (I. Clausen 2007, pers. comm.). The age difference of over 3000 years between the fish and the charcoal from Kayhude is much larger than the reservoir ages that we find for modern fish, but of the same order of magnitude as the reservoir age for modern water and plants. None of the food crusts are as old as the fishbones, though. The humic fraction of two food crusts has also been dated (Table 1.3). The humic fraction is likely to consist of humic acids from the soil, and is thus removed from the samples. Here it is older than the food crusts (Figure 1.3), indicating contamination with an older soil substance.

The hardwater effect at Schlamersdorf and Kayhude seems to be larger than the effect reported by Fischer and Heinemeier (2003), at least for the fishbones. In their study area, the Åmose on Zealand, Denmark, the fish was 100 to 500 ^{14}C years older than the archaeological context, while the food crusts were up to 300 ^{14}C years older.

Conclusion and future plans

According to our results, a reservoir effect of between a few hundred and a few thousand years seems possible in the pottery from Schlamersdorf and Kayhude. The large variability in ages leads to a high variability in the estimated reservoir age and thus to a broad range of the estimated 'real' age of the pottery of, for example, 5300 to 4500 BC. The dating of 4750 BC for coastal Ertebølle pottery is most likely too old as its $\delta^{13}C$ value of -20‰ indicates a large marine component (Hartz and Lübke 2006), and we assume a later introduction of pottery to the coastal sites of Schleswig-Holstein. The pottery from these inland sites can thus be older, equally old or even younger than the pottery from coastal sites.

With the broad age range for the oldest pottery in Schleswig-Holstein, several cultures come into consideration as the source of this innovation. Import finds show connections between the Ertebølle culture and fully Neolithic cultures to the south and east of the river Elbe (cf. Hartz and Glykou 2008), which are a possible source of ceramic knowledge. Interestingly, other Late Mesolithic groups throughout northern Europe produced pottery, often quite similar to the typical pointed-based pots of the Ertebølle culture (see Table 1.4), so that the origin of Ertebølle pottery is not necessarily a Neolithic culture. The eastern Baltic (pottery from around 5000 BC), or the Netherlands and Belgium (from around 4700 BC) could have been the regions of origin.

The stable isotope ratios $\delta^{13}C$ and $\delta^{15}N$ are only suitable to a limited extent for identification of the ingredients of a food crust. The hardwater effect can lead to varying and possibly very high ^{14}C age offsets. Thus, ^{14}C dates of such samples should be treated with extreme caution. Radiocarbon dating of the experimental food crusts is in progress. We hope to find a correlation between the stable isotope values and the ^{14}C age of a certain sample of a food crust.

Ertebølle Cuisine

Table 1.4. Examples of hunter-gatherer pottery in northern Europe. Some authors define the beginning of the Neolithic as the beginning of pottery production, not as the beginning of agriculture. The cultures characterized as 'Neolithic' in this table were also hunter-gatherer cultures. Where only ^{14}C ages BP were given, I calibrated them with OxCal 4.1, using the calibration curve IntCal09, and put the 95.4% age ranges in brackets (see text for references).

Site(s)/ Region	Culture/Group	Age/Period	Description	References
Hüde I am Dümmer (NW Germany)		4200–3700 BC (uncalibrated)	'large vessels with pointed bases, very similar to those of the Ertebølle/Ellerbek culture of the Baltic area'	Bogucki, P. 1988. *Forest farmers and stockherders*, Cambridge
Osa (Latvia)	'Early Neolithic'	5730±50 BP 5580±80 BP 5780±70 BP (4692–4460 BC 4608–4262 BC 4788–4464 BC)	'…large, thick-walled pots with pointed bottoms and […] small, ovoid 'lamps'. The pottery is ornamented with comb stamps, lines and small pits, forming horizontal or diagonal rows or zig-zag patterns.'	Dolukhanov, P.M. and Liiva, A.A. 1979. 'Prehistoric Civilizations in the Baltic Basin', in Gudelis V. and Königsson, L.-K. (eds.), *The Quaternary History of the Baltic*, Uppsala, 243–249.
Särnate (Latvia)		4045–2496 BC (my calibration; extremes of 94.5% ranges from 5 datings)	'conical vessels with straight or S-shaped rims and small 'lamps''	Dolukhanov and Liiva 1979 (see above)
Åland	Early Older Comb Ware Culture	around 5000 BC; pottery from the same culture in Finland and Karelia, Russia: 5400–4200 BC	'un-profiled pots with a round or pointed bottom', tempered with crushed rock, sometimes with sand, surface often decorated (cords, stamps)	Hallgren, F. 2004. 'The introduction of ceramic technology around the Baltic Sea in the 6th millennium', in Knuttson, H. (ed.), *Proceedings of the Final Coast to Coast Conference 1–5 Oct. 2002 in Falköping, Sweden*, Uppsala, 123–142.
Eastern Baltic	Narva Culture	'…it should be safe to conclude that pottery appears around 5500–5200 cal BC in the Narva Culture.'	'large pots with pointed base and low plates, very reminiscent of the Erteböll clay lamps… The richly decorated Erteböll vessels display clear similarities to Narva pottery…'	Hallgren 2004 (see above)

Site(s)/ Region	Culture/Group	Age/Period	Description	References
NE Poland, S Lithuania, SW Byelorussia	Neman Culture	Neman datings from Poland: 5900±100 BP, 5700±120 BP (5030–4529 BC, 4827–4335 BC) from Lithuania: 6550, 6020, 5980, 5950, 5360, all ±70 BP (the oldest: 5623–5374 BC)	vessels have slightly profiled shape and pointed bottoms	Hallgren 2004 (see above)
Melsele-Hof ten Damme (NW Belgium)	Rhine-Meuse-Schelde-Culture	Mesolithic, although remains from domesticated cattle and pigs were found	'The potsherds are tempered with schamotte, bone and quartz and show pointed base vessels and sparse decoration'	Heinen, M. 2006. 'The Rhine-Meuse-Schelde Culture in *Western Europe. Distribution, Chronology and Development*', in Kind, C.-J. (ed.), *After the Ice Age. Settlements, subsistence and social development on the Mesolithic of Central Europe*, Stuttgart, 75–86.
W Europe, Baltic		Mesolithic	pointed-based pottery is a characteristic trait of a range of subneolithic and mesolithic cultures along the whole of the Atlantic fringe and further to the east in the Baltic	Klassen, L. 2002. 'The Ertebølle Culture and Neolithic Continental Europe traces of contact and interaction', in Fischer, A. and Kristiansen K. (eds.), *The Neolithization of Denmark. 150 years of debate*, Sheffield, 305–317.
Dabki 9, Baltic coast of Pommerania		6300–5300 BP (cal. 95.4% age range of 6800±500 BP: 6909–4621 BC)	'…Mesolithic flints, rich pottery collection of Ertebølle type with an admixture of Linear Ceramic pottery, […] and especially a growing number of bones from cattle and pigs.'	Kobusiewicz, M. 2006. 'Paraneolithic – Obstinate Hunter-Gatherers of the Polish Plain', in Kind, C.-J. (ed.), *After the Ice Age. Settlements, subsistence and social development on the Mesolithic of Central Europe*, Stuttgart, 181–188.

Ertebølle Cuisine

Site(s)/ Region	Culture/Group	Age/Period	Description	References
Swifterbant, Netherlands	Early Neolithic	around 3300 BC	'…pottery in a Nordic (Ertebølle) style and (trade) relationships with late Rössen communities…'	Louwe-Kooijmans, L.P. 1980. 'Archaeology and Coastal Change in the Netherlands', in Thompson, F.H. (ed.), *Archaeology and coastal change*, London, 106–133.
Polderweg, Netherlands		4700 BC	'Op de site Polderweg werd alleen in het hoogste niveau (4700 v. Chr.) een beperkt aantal aardewerkscherven gevonden, waaronder een karakteristiek dikwandig kommetje met puntbodem.'	Louwe-Kooijmans, L.P. 1998. 'Trijntje van de Betuweroute, jachtkampen uit de Steentijd te Hardinxveld-Giessendam', *Spiegel Historiael* 33, 423–428.
Swifterbant S2 and S3, Netherlands	Early Neolithic	3400–3200 BC 'The C14 dates correspond to the initial phases of the Michelsberg culture (Germany, Belgium) and the end of the Ertebølle culture (Denmark, northern Germany)'	'…pots with a flowing S-shaped profile and round or pointed bases'	de Roever, J.P. 1979. 'The pottery from Swifterbant – Dutch Ertebølle?' *Helinium* 19, 13–36.
Doel 'Deurganckdok', Belgium	Final Swifterbant) Mesolithic	food crusts 4900–4700 BC, carbonized plant/bone: 4500–4000 BC	'…dominated by slightly S-shaped vessels, provided with a rounded or pointed base'	Sergant, J., Crombé, P. and Perdaen, Y. 2006. 'The Sites of Doel 'Deurganckdok' and the Mesolithic/Neolithic Transition in the Sandy Lowlands of Belgium', in Guilane and v. Berg (eds), *La Néolithisation / The Neolithization Process*, Oxford, 53–60.

Acknowledgements

This work would not have been possible without the contributions from the following colleagues, and we would like to thank them all: Sönke Hartz and Ingo Clausen for providing us with the archaeological samples; Sönke Hartz, Harm Paulsen, Aikaterini Glykou and Mara Weber for their help and company during the food crust experiments; the Århus AMS group, Klaus Bahner, Claus Grosen, Hanne Jakobsen, Ann Berith Jensen, Vibeke Jensen, for help with the sample pretreatment and measurement; Claus von Carnap-Bornheim for financing thirty of the datings and the Prof. Werner Petersen-Stiftung Foundation in Kiel, Germany, for providing the funds; and finally Hans van der Plicht for very useful comments on the first version of this manuscript.

References

Ambrose, S.H. 2001. 'Controlled Diet and Climate Experiments on Nitrogen Isotope Ratios of Rats', in Ambrose, S.H. (ed.), *Biogeochemical Approaches in Paleodietary Analysis*, New York, 243–259.

Andersen, G.J., Heinemeier, J., Nielsen, H.L., Rud, N., Thomsen, M.S., Johnsen, S., Sveinbjörnsdóttir, Á. and Hjartarson, Á. 1989. 'AMS ^{14}C dating on the Fossvogur sediments, Iceland', *Radiocarbon* 31(3), 592–600.

Arneborg, J., Heinemeier J., Lynnerup, N., Nielsen, H.L., Rud, N. and Sveinbjörnsdottir, Á.E. 1999. 'Change of Diet of the Greenland Vikings Determined from Stable Carbon Isotope Analysis and ^{14}C Dating of Their Bones', *Radiocarbon* 41(2), 157–168.

Boaretto, E., Thorling, L., Sveinbjörnsdóttir, A.E., Yechieli, Y. and Heinemeier, J. 1998. 'Study of the effect of fossil organic carbon on ^{14}C in groundwater from Hvinningdal, Denmark', *Radiocarbon* 40(2), 915–920.

Boudin, M., Strydonck, M.V. and Crombé, P. In press. 'Radiocarbon Dating of Pottery Food Crusts: Reservoir Effect or Not? The Case of Swifterbant Pottery from Doel 'Deurganckdok' (Belgium)', in Crombé, P., Strydonck, M.V., Sergant, M., Boudin, M. and Bats, M. (eds.), *Chronology and Evolution in the Mesolithic of North-West Europe*, Newcastle upon Tyne, 753–772.

Bronk Ramsey, C. 2009. 'Bayesian analysis of radiocarbon dates', *Radiocarbon* 51(1), 337–360.

Brown, T.A., Nelson, D.E., Vogel, J.S. and Southon, J.R. 1988. 'Improved collagen extraction by improved Longin method', *Radiocarbon* 30(2), 171–177.

Clark, I.D. and Fritz, P. 1997. *Environmental Isotopes in Hydrogeology*, New York.

Clausen, I. 2008. 'Von späten Jägern und frühen Bauern. Binnen-ländische Ertebølle-Kultur bei Kayhude, Kreis Segeberg', *Archäologische Nachrichten aus Schleswig-Holstein* 14, 14–16.

Cook, G.T., Bonsall, C., Hedges, R.E.M., McSweeney, K., Boroneanţ, V. and Pettit, P.B. 2001. 'A Freshwater Diet-Derived ^{14}C Reservoir Effect at the Stone Age Sites in the Iron Gates Gorge;, *Radiocarbon* 43(2A), 453–460.

Craig, H. 1957. 'Isotopic standards for carbon and oxygen and correction factors for mass-spectrometric analyses of carbon dioxide', *Geochimica et Cosmochimica Acta* 12(1–2), 133–149.

Deevey, E.S., Gross, M.S., Hutchinson, G.E. and Kraybill, H.L. 1954. 'The Natural C14 Contents of Materials from Hard-Water Lakes', *PNAS – Proceedings of the National Academy of Sciences of the United States of America* 40, 285–288.

Fischer, A. and Heinemeier, J. 2003. 'Freshwater Reservoir Effect in ^{14}C Dates of Food Residue on Pottery', *Radiocarbon* 45(3), 449–466.

Fontes, J.-C. and Garnier, J.-M. 1979. 'Determination of the initial ^{14}C activity of total dissolved carbon', *Water Resources Research* 15(2), 399–413.

Godwin, H. 1951. 'Comments on radiocarbon dating samples from the British Isles', *American Journal of Science* 249, 301–307.

Hartz, S. 1993. 'Inland-Ertebølle in Schleswig-Holstein. Die Fundstelle Schlamersdorf LA5, Kr. Stormarn', in Meier, D. (ed.), *Archäologie in Schleswig 1/1991 [Symposium Wohlde]* Kiel, 33–38.

Hartz, S. 1996. 'Zehnter Arbeitsbericht des Archäologischen Landesamtes Schleswig-Holstein. Grabungsberichte der Jahre 1988–1993: Travenbrück Altgemeinde Schlamersdorf, Kr. Stormarn, Steinzeitliche Wohnplätze Travenbrück, LA5 und LA15', *Offa* 53, 374–378.

Hartz, S. 1997. 'Ertebøllekultur im Travetal. Ausgrabungen auf dem Fundplatz Travenbrück LA 5 Gemarkung Schlamersdorf, Kreis Stormarn. Ein Vorbericht', *Stormarner Hefte* 20, 171–186.

Hartz, S. and Lübke, H. 2006. 'New Evidence for a Chronostratigraphic Division of the Ertebølle Culture and the Earliest Funnel Beaker Culture on the Southern Mecklenburg Bay', in Kind, C.-J. (ed.), *After the Ice Age. Settlements, subsistence and social development on the Mesolithic of Central Europe.* Stuttgart, 59–74.

Hartz, S. and Glykou, A. 2008. 'Neues aus Neustadt: Ausgrabungen zur Ertebølle- und frühen Trichterbecher-Kultur in Schleswig-Holstein', *Archäologische Nachrichten aus Schleswig-Holstein* 14, 17–19.

Heier-Nielsen, S., Heinemeier, J., Nielsen, H.L. and Rud, N. 1995. 'Recent Reservoir Ages for Danish Fjords and Marine Waters', *Radiocarbon* 37(3), 875–882.

Jørkov, M.L.S., Heinemeier, J. and Lynnerup, N. 2007. 'Evaluating bone collagen extraction methods for stable isotope analysis in dietary studies', *Journal of Archaeological Science* 34(11), 1824–1829.

Kanstrup, M. 2008. *Madkultur – vane og variation. Koststudier baseret på isotopanalyser af skeletmateriale fra vikingetidsgravpladsen Galgedil på Nordfyn*, Konferencespeciale, Afdeling for forhistorisk arkæologi, Aarhus Universitet.

Lanting, J.N. and van der Plicht, J. 1995/1996. 'Wat hebben Floris V, skelet swifterbant S2 en visotters gemeen?' *Palaeohistoria* 37/38, 491–519.

Longin, R. 1971. 'New method of collagen extraction for radiocarbon dating', *Nature* 230, 241–242.

Mariotti, A. 1983. 'Atmospheric nitrogen is a reliable standard for natural ^{15}N abundance measurements', *Nature* 303(5919), 685–687

Olsen, J., Heinemeier, J., Lübcke, H., Lüth, F. and Terberger, T. 2010. 'Dietary habits and freshwater reservoir effects in bones from a Neolithic Northern German cemetery', *Radiocarbon* 52(2–3), 635–644.

Olsson, I.U. 1976. *The importance of the pretreatment of wood and charcoal samples*, Radiocarbon dating – ninth international conference, Los Angeles and La Jolla.

Philippsen, B. 2010. 'Die älteste Keramik', *Archäologische Nachrichten aus Schleswig-Holstein* 2009 15, 52–55.

Reimer, P.J., Baillie, M.G.L., et al. 2009. 'IntCal09 and Marine09 Radiocarbon Age Calibration Curves, 0–50,000 Years cal BP', *Radiocarbon* 51(4), 1111–1150.

Schoeninger, M.J., DeNiro, M.-J. and Tauber, H. 1983. 'Stable nitrogen isotope ratios of bone collagen reflect marine and terrestrial components of prehistoric human diet', *Science* 220, 1381–1383.

Smits, L. and van der Plicht, H. 2009. 'Mesolithic and Neolithic human remains in the Netherlands: physical anthropological and stable isotope investigations', *Journal of Archaeology in the Low Countries* 1(1), 55–85.

Stuiver, M. and Polach, H.A. 1977. 'Discussion. Reporting of ^{14}C Data', *Radiocarbon* 19(3), 355–363.

Tauber, H. 1979. '^{14}C Activity of Arctic Marine Mammals', 9th International Radiocarbon Conference, Los Angeles and La Jolla, Berkeley.

Fun and Feasting: Contextualizing the Animal Remains from the Kabeirion at Thebes

Kirsten Bedigan
University of Glasgow

The animal remains from the sanctuary of Kabeiroi near Thebes present a relatively comprehensive corpus of material from a single religious complex occupied from the sixth century BC until the fourth century AD. The sanctuary is dedicated to deities of whom relatively little is known compared with other gods in the Greek pantheon. The Kabeiroi are identified as a father and son pairing (Kabeiros and Pais) who have associations with agricultural, pastoral and human fertility (Bedigan 2008, 43). Issues arising during and after the excavations led to complications with the publication of findings (Bedigan 2008, 47–49). Originally the animal remains should have been published as part of the main series of excavation reports *Das Kabirenheiligtum bei Theben* (see Schmaltz 1974, n.p.; Heyder and Mallwitz 1978, vi). Their presentation independently means that the relationship between the cult centre and two categories of bone finds (dedications and food debris) has been harder to identify – a situation hindered by the absence of find contexts in Boessneck's report (1973). This paper will discuss the animal remains from the site and consider them in conjunction with the architecture and votive offerings at the sanctuary.

The animal remains: an overview
Analysis of the remains clearly indicates that there were trends in the species found at the sanctuary. The patterns of consumption stayed relatively stable. The remains present at the site encompass both domesticated and wild species. The animals not associated with food consumption or sacrifice (such as foxes, frogs, etc.) suggests that a small proportion of the remains represent accidental interment rather than anything associated with the cult (Boessneck 1973, 28). The majority of the finds, with the anomalies excluded, constitute species which are edible. Chronologically, the finds are present for most of the sanctuary's lifespan, although some phases lack material – whether this is due to an absence of faunal remains or a lack of dating evidence is unclear. The totals for the most frequent species (primarily sheep/goat, cattle and deer) indicate a fluctuating picture with peaks in the main Hellenistic and Roman period, but a decrease in the intervening period (Figure 2.1; Boessneck 1973, 3–6, tables 2–6). The subsequent decline in animal remains after 350 AD corresponds with the other archaeological evidence as the site shows decreased activity prior to its abandonment in the late fourth–fifth centuries AD (Boessneck 1973, 6, table 6; Bedigan 2008, 400, 404–406).

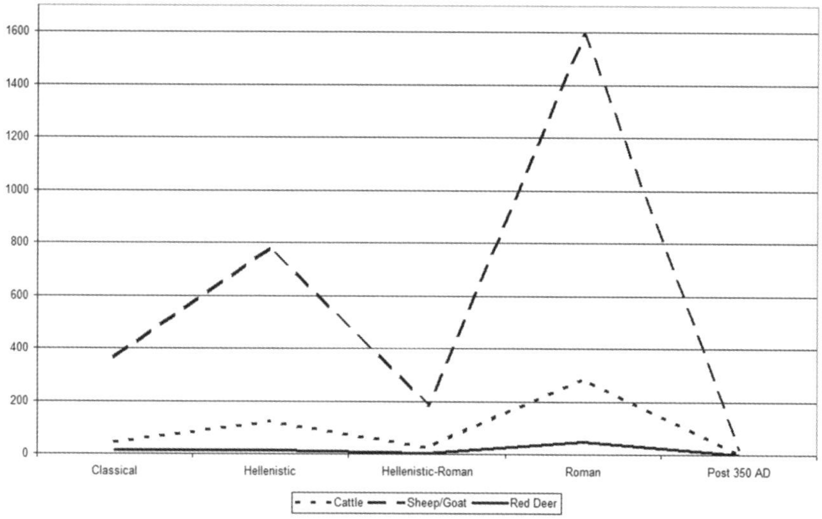

Figure 2.1. Chronological distribution for cattle, sheep/goats and red deer at the Kabeirion (based on Boessneck 1973, 3–6, tables 2–6).

Attempts to determine the age and gender of the remains at the site yield limited results. This data is not available for many species and given the poor condition of many of the finds this is not unexpected (Boessneck 1973, 1). Summarizing the published information we can make some tentative conclusions (Table 2.1). Firstly, both male and female animals are offered at the sanctuary. However, the bones indicate that there were more males present (Schmaltz 1980, 13). Secondly, age categories vary. Those species with a small number of finds tend to yield more remains and are described as young. The larger samples provide a more complete picture and clearly demonstrate that animals of all ages were present in the archaeological record. Both the cattle and sheep/goat categories offer a fairly similar distribution of ages, approximately one-third of the remains are from infants/juveniles, with the other two-thirds from sub-adults/adults (Boessneck 1973, 11, 15 table 10).

Specific find contexts are not available as these were omitted from the publication of the remains as it made the material unwieldy (Boessneck 1973, 1). From the extant information, it appears that a significant proportion of the bones were located in two distinct deposits. None of the other archaeological features revealed in the excavations have references to animal remains being found in their vicinity. According to Schachter (1986, 108 n.1) the majority of the remains were located in one of the two sacrificial pits located behind the so-called 'Temple 1' excavated during the original investigation in 1887–1888 (see also Wolters and Bruns 1940, 3). Initial reports on the pits only claim that a large number of goat or sheep metatarsal bones were excavated here (Wolters and Bruns 1940, 3; Hemberg 1950, 197 n.3). Subsequent excavations in 1959 and 1962 yielded ceramics datable to the fifth century BC (Bruns 1963, 115; Bruns 1964, 239,

241–242 fig.8). However, the majority of bone material from the sanctuary dates to the Hellenistic period or later (Boessneck 1973, 3–8, tables 2–8). It seems unlikely therefore, that this is the largest concentration of finds from the site as a whole, rather it is the largest sample known with both find context and relative date.

Table 2.1. Estimated gender and age categories for all species excavated at the sanctuary (based on Boessneck 1973).

Species	Total	Gender			Age Category						
		♂	♀	?	Infant	Juv-enile	Sub-Adult	Sub-Adult / Adult	Adult	Mature	?
Cattle	530	•	•		•	•	•	•	•		
Sheep/ Goat	3238	•	•		•	•	•	•	•		
Pig	47			•		•	•	•	•		•
Horse/ Donkey	3			•							•
Dog	3			•	•	•					•
Chicken	6										
Pigeon, Domestic	1			•		•					•
Red Deer	69	•	•								•
Fallow Deer	14		•	•							•
Roe Deer	25			•							•
Red Fox	4			•							•
Hare	36			•			•				•
Mole Rat	3			•							•
Bird, Unknown	4			•			•				•
Mallard	2			•							•
Pigeon, Wood	2			•							•
Coot	1			•							•
Buzzard	1			•							•
Owl, Little	2			•							•
Tortoise	12			•			•				•
Marsh Frog	1			•							•
Unknown	800	-	-	-	-	-	-	-	-	-	-

Fun and Feasting

The other location is the building 'Middle Tholos 18', the excavated contents included ash and charcoal layers containing animal bones and ceramic vessels (Wolters and Bruns 1940, 3; Heyder and Mallwitz 1978, 44–47; Cooper and Morris 1990, 66). No specifics are available on the species/types of bones found. The finds indicate that this structure, along with other similar buildings, was used for the consumption of food and beverages which formed part of the rituals (Cooper and Morris 1990, 66; Batino 2004, 197). The finds are associated with an *eschara* at the centre of the tholos, a sacred hearth comprising a pit ringed with stones, which is perhaps indicative of cooking within the structure (Bruns 1967, 232; Lehmann 1998, 77; Evans 2002, 236 n.17).

References to other faunal remains are known, a set of three fourth-century BC sacrificial pits were located in the vicinity of the niche structure in the Roman retaining wall. The first was connected to an adjoining gutter, the second contained ash, and the third was said to be used for meat and bones (Bruns 1967, 264). The 'Lower Tholos 12' also had ash deposits, analysis of these failed to confirm the presence of organic residues although Bruns (1963, 117) did not rule out the possibility of ash being derived from animal remains. Other bone fragments have been located in reused fill for foundation deposits (Wolters and Bruns 1940, 4).

The votive offerings: knucklebones

Knucklebones, or *astragaloi*, comprise approximately one-fifth of the overall total of recovered animal remains (Boessneck 1973, 1). Their frequency is not surprising given the popularity of these gaming pieces as dedications (Parlama and Stampolidis 2001, 302 no.297). It is clear that these finds represent a distinct group of animal remains

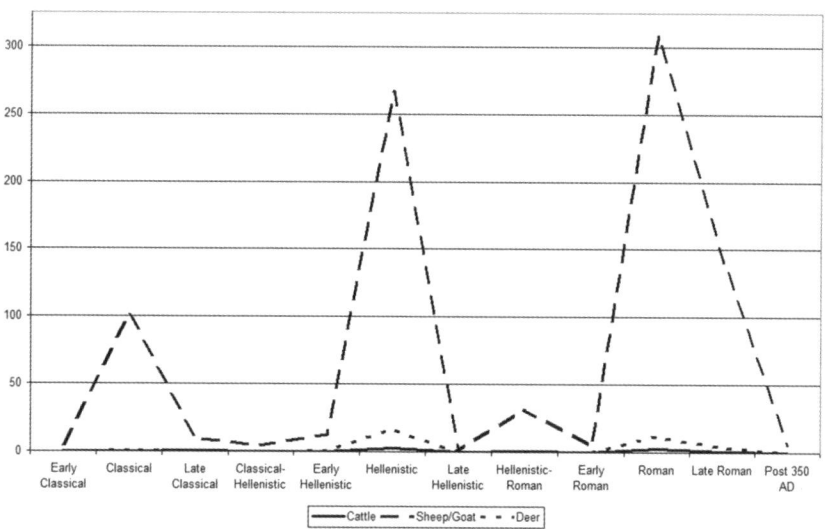

Figure 2.2. Chronological distribution for cattle, sheep/goat and deer (red, fallow and roe) knucklebones at the Kabeirion (based on Boessneck 1973, 8, table 8).

and must be considered separately for accurate conclusions to be drawn. The patterns of dedication for these follow the chronological trends displayed by the other animal remains (Figure 2.2; Boessneck 1973, 8, table 2.8).

It can be suggested that the knucklebones are obtained from animals offered as sacrifices (Bruns 1963, 121; Bruns 1964, 262). The proportions of knucklebones by species would reflect the overall picture of animal remains quite closely with the majority from sheep/goats, with low numbers of cattle and deer. A significant proportion of the knucklebones were processed, either by sanding specific sides of the bone or by drilling holes (see Table 2.2; Boessneck 1973, 9–10). This type of processing may have taken place elsewhere before the knucklebones were deposited at the site.

There are also a number of other non-organic astragaloi which have been manufactured for dedication in a variety of materials including stone, metal, glass and amber (Table 2.2). The presence of these finds in other fabrics argues strongly that knucklebones were an accepted dedication and that they were connected to the cult in this role rather than a product of sacrifice (Reese 1989, 64; Parlama and Stampolidis 2000, 302 no.297). Bruns (1963, 121; 1964, 262) believes that the popularity of knucklebones as a game for children, and their presence at the site was connected to the deity *Pais,* 'the child', a worthy recipient of a typical childhood game (Schachter 2003, 122). This hypothesis can be strengthened by the dedication of other toys at the sanctuary (Bruns 1964, 262; Bedigan 2008, 122–123). The concept that they were dedications is strengthened by the dimensions of some examples, as larger knucklebones would inhibit game play. One example, a bronze *astragalos,* measures 40–60mm long and 8mm thick (Wolters 1890b, 376). Those from the larger animals are comparable in size to the aforementioned bronze example. The sheep/goat knucklebones tend to be more usable, measuring 25–35mm long (Boessneck 1973, pl. 1–2).

Consumption
Evidence for sacrifice
There is a belief that every bone found at a sanctuary is evidence of sacrifice, yet food consumption is not confined to those animals that were offered to the gods (Reese 2005, 123). The animal species associated with sacrifice are domesticated (Burkert 2001, 55), with sheep and goats as the preferred offering. The function of the non-domesticated species at the Kabeirion are harder to determine, they may be anomalous deposits or be derived from hunting/sacrifice (Boessneck 1973, 28).

Animal sacrifice involved the burning of selected parts of the victim. This included the inner organs, the bones and other inedible remains (Burkert 2001, 56–57; Gilhus 2006, 115). The meat was cooked and consumed by the participants as part of a public distribution ritual (Symons 2002, 434, 443; Gilhus 2006, 116). The evidence for burning in relation to the Kabeirion finds is limited. A number of knucklebones mentioned by Boessneck (1973, 10) are described as being charred or calcinated. The other remains have no references to burning (Boessneck 1973). However, the lack of gender

Table 2.2. Fabric, species (where appropriate) and processing information for the knucklebones based upon the archaeological and epigraphic evidence (Dittenberger 1892: No.2420; Wolters 1890b: 375–376; Bruns 1963: 121; Bruns 1964: 262; Archaeological Museum, Thebes; Ure Museum, Reading).

Fabric		Totals	Processed	Unprocessed
Bone	Cattle	12	2	10
	Sheep/Goat	933	282	651
	Red Deer	11	6	5
	Fallow Deer	11	7	4
	Roe Deer	20	1	19
	Unknown	2	-	-
Glass	-	1 +	-	-
Stone	Steatite (Soapstone)	2 +	-	-
	Other	3 +	-	-
Amber	-	1 +	-	-
Metal	Lead	1 +	-	-
	Bronze	2 +	-	-
	Silver	4 +	-	-

determination for cattle may be a result of the bones being burned (Reese 2005, 123). Reese (2005, 123) also confirms that the deer bones are not burnt, suggesting hunting rather than sacrifice.

There are numerous representations of animals at the Kabeirion, in terracotta and metal, and on vases (Bruns 1959, 246), with bulls proving the most popular (Schachter 1986, 107). Chronologically, the metal figurines are dated to the tenth–fifth centuries BC with the terracottas appearing in the fifth–fourth centuries BC (Schachter 1986, 91 n.3). The terracotta animal figurines are currently unpublished (Schmaltz 1980, 160 n.397; Schachter 2003, 126–127). Approximate totals can be obtained and indicate that a variety of species were available as figurines (Table 2.3).

There are several debates as to the purpose of these figurines and vases, especially as to whether they had a symbolic function (Lembesi 1993, 2). Firstly, the bull figurines may have personified the ideal sacrifice (Schachter 2003, 139 n.12). The ancient texts strongly suggest that cattle were the premier animal for sacrifice (Bevan 1986, 82). However, Lembesi (1993, 18) and Daumas (2003, 138) both argue that these bull figurines cannot represent sacrificial animals as the statuettes depict adult animals while the bones are primarily juvenile. However, the assertion relating to the predominance of juveniles is likely to be due to a mistranslation of Boessneck's report (1973, 11) where it is clear that two-thirds of the cattle identified at the site were adult. The conclusions drawn by Lembesi (1993, 10) and Daumas (2003, 140) argue that the bull figurines

Table 2.3. Approximate totals for the metal and terracotta animal figurines from the sanctuary (Hemberg 1950, 186–7; Lembesi 1993, 18; Wolters 1890a: 356–358).

Figurine Type	Metal	Terracotta
Bull	534	600 +
Sheep	8 +	+/- 250
Goat	10 +	+/- 50
Pig	-	200 +
Dog	-	20
Hare	-	6
Lion	-	+/- 25
Cockerel	-	+/- 36
Other Birds	-	+/- 25
Other Animals	-	?

represented the completion of a coming-of-age ritual (see Barringer 2001, 13). There are a large number of figurines of youths (standing with a ram, lyre, pillar, cockerel or dove, in various forms of dress) which Daumas (2003, 140) used to support these claims (for a full catalogue of the figurines, see Schmaltz 1974). The third interpretation regarding the purpose of these bulls is that they were connected with herdsmen invoking divine protection for their livestock (Schachter 1986, 97). The presence of bull figurines at other sites in the vicinity of the Kabeirion and Thebes can be used in support of this argument (Schachter 1986, 97 n.1).

Bulls are also depicted on a number of the vases from the site. Interestingly they are not always associated with scenes relating to sacrifice. There is only one confirmed scene where the bull is being presented as a sacrifice, and in that instance is being presented to a herm (Wolters and Bruns 1940, 101, fig.4, pl. 51.5–6; Braun and Haevernick 1981, 66 no.389). Other images show Kabeiros and a bull posed together, indicating that the two are linked (Wolters and Bruns 1940, 96, pl. 6; Braun and Haevernick 1981, 62 no.297). Daumas (2003, 141) argues that this particular scene may show worshippers approaching the cult statue as the divine figure is larger than life-size. This is purely conjecture as gods and statues are normally depicted on a greater scale (Van Straten 1995, 170). The bull and god pairing is commonly found elsewhere in ancient Greece and indicates a strong connection to Dionysus (Bevan 1986, 83, 95). The iconography from the Kabeirion is clearly Dionysiac in nature (Bedigan 2008, 289–293). The remaining vases are fragmentary and tend to only preserve characteristic elements of the bull (horns, legs etc.) without any context as to what the scene may have been.

There is a lack of correlation between bones and images found at the sanctuary. If we were to interpret the animal remains, we would expect a greater proportion of sheep and goat figurines rather than bulls. This is not unusual. While the available literature states that cattle were the primary choice for sacrifice, the number of cattle bones found at sanctuaries is low (Bevan 1986, 82, 86). It seems likely that the variation between the animals offered for sacrifice and the figurines related to expenditure. Different offerings reflect the costs involved (Bruns 1959, 246). Bulls are an expensive offering (Schachter 2003, 126–127) whereas a sheep or goat, or a terracotta/metal figurine is more accessible to a far wider range of participants.

Evidence for other food consumption
Although linked directly to the animals sacrificed and consumed at the sanctuary as part of the offerings to the gods, there is evidence to suggest that other animal remains were consumed at the sanctuary as a separate category (Gilhus 2006, 17). The lack of burning on the deer bones clearly indicates that they were not offered to the Kabeiroi as a sacrifice as we would define it (Reese 2005, 123). Supply from hunting is not guaranteed, and the wild remains at the site are presumably occasional offerings rather than a standard practice (Bevan 1986, 104–105; Symons 2002, 441). The value of the remains as trophies worthy of dedication may be connected to hunting as a means of demonstrating the social importance of the dedicating hunter(s) (Hamilakis 2003, 240). This is perhaps supported by the absence of deer figurines – it was not an animal normally associated with the Kabeiroi.

Conclusions

The two categories of animal remains – votives and food consumption (Boessneck 1973, 1) – can be further refined. The debris from feasting at the site can be sub-divided into those animals which were eaten as part of a sacrifice and those who were not. The increase in bones from edible animals in the Hellenistic and Roman periods does correspond with quantitative increases of other evidence at the sanctuary for those phases (Heyder and Mallwitz 1978, 62–69; Schachter 1986, 81–88). Architecturally the development of the site from the Hellenistic period onwards shows the expansion of structures specifically designed for dining and drinking (Heyder and Mallwitz 1978, 40–43, 51–53, 54–56; Schachter 1986, 81–88, esp. 87–88). The stoas to the south/south-west of the sanctuary provided more space for participants during and after the Hellenistic period.

The lack of correlation between the types of bones found and the votives at the sanctuary is connected to these participants. Dedications vary depending on a number of circumstances: the people offering them, the purpose for which they were offered and the occasion when they were given all impact on the dedication itself (Antonaccio 2005, 101). Costs also play a role in this. According to Antonaccio (2005, 101), cattle are the most expensive offering and would be associated with grand occasions, presumably events like annual festivals involving a large number of people. Sheep (and goats) are effectively in the middle price range and would be sacrificed by communal groups such as the *polis* whereas pigs are the cheapest option and represent sacrifices by family groups or individuals (Van Straten 1995, 176–177; Antonaccio 2005, 101). If we apply the above hypothesis to the evidence from the Kabeirion we would reach the conclusion that the majority of sacrifices were offered by the community. However, we lack evidence that the Kabeirion had a large annual festival (although it would seem unlikely that there was no such event) which would presumably represent the type of occasion when cattle would be an appropriate sacrifice. This theory also fails to consider the possible variables, such as the wealth of the individual/family. Those with greater socioeconomic means are likely to offer valuable dedications or sacrifices as a method of accepted public display of status and wealth (Becker, 97). The votive figurines of animals do not need to relate to sacrificial practices, although they can act as a substitute if circumstances dictate (Bevan 1986, 320, 322; Antonaccio 2005, 100). The presence of lion figurines at the sanctuary does support the premise that the votives did not necessarily reflect sacrificial practices. The Kabeiroi, like other Greek deities, could receive figurines of a variety of species (Bevan 1986, 320). The prominence of domesticated animals in the extant figurines, with the exception of boars and lions, would suggest that the dedicators were seeking protection or fertility for their herds and flocks (Bevan 1986, 322, 328).

It can be said that the animal remains at the Kabeirion are comparable to those of other Greek sanctuaries. There is a definable relationship between the bones, the other votives and the architecture. The bones indicate that there was an active system of sacrifice of domesticated animals at the site which probably involved the local *polis*, and that these animals were supplemented by other wild species. The figurines demonstrate preferences for certain species, with a clear emphasis (if we exclude the lions) for domesticated animals and suggests that they could substitute sacrifice and acting as a plea or token of gratitude on the part of the community.

Acknowledgements

This research was facilitated through the Tytus Summer Residency Fellowship awarded by the Department of Classics and the Burnam Classics Library at University of Cincinnati. I would like to thank the following for their help: Anne Wilde, Naomi Sykes, my colleagues at the University of Glasgow, the University of Cincinnati and the Burnam Classics Library, and JM and JB.

References

Antonaccio, C.M. 2005. 'Dedications and the character of cult', in Hägg, R. and Alroth, B. (eds.), *Greek Sacrificial Ritual, Olympian and Chthonian. Proceedings of the Sixth International Seminar on Ancient Greek Cult*, Stockholm, 121–123.

Barringer, J.M. 2001. *The Hunt in Ancient Greece*, Baltimore and London.

Batino, S. 2004. '"Tholos: Peripheres Oikodomina": Considerazioni su "Rundbau" e "Rechteckbau" nel Kabirion Tebano', *Annuario della Scuola archeologica di Atene e delle Missioni italiane in Oriente* 82, 195–208.

Becker, H. 2009. 'The economic agency of the Etruscan temple: elites, dedications and display', in Gleba, M. and Becker, H. (eds.), *Votives, Places and Rituals in Etruscan Religion: Studies in Honor of Jean MacIntosh Turfa*, Leiden, 87–100.

Bedigan, K.M. 2008. *Boeotian Kabeiric Ware: The Significance of the Ceramic Offerings at the Theban Kabeirion in Boeotia*, University of Glasgow, Unpublished PhD Thesis.

Bevan, E. 1986. *Representations of Animals in Sanctuaries of Artemis and other Olympian Deities*, Oxford.

Boessneck, J. 1973. *Die Tierknochenfunde aus dem Kabirenheiligtum bei Theben (Böotien)*, Munich.
Braun, K. and Haevernick, T.E. 1981. *Bemalte Keramik und Glas aus dem Kabirenheiligtum bei Theben*, Berlin.
Bruns, G. 1959. 'Die Ausgrabungen im Kabirenheiligtum bei Theben in Böotien', in Deutsches Archäologisches Institut, *Neue Deutsche Ausgrabungen um Mittelmeer gebiet und im Vorderen Orient*, Berlin, 237–248.
Bruns, G. 1963. 'Grabungen im Kabirenheiligtum bei Theben', *Archaiologikon Deltion* 18, 115–121.
Bruns, G. 1964. 'Kabirenheiligtum bei Theben. Vorläufiger bericht über die Grabungskampagnen 1959 und 1962', *Archäologischer Anzeiger* 79, 231–265.
Bruns, G. 1967. 'Kabirenheiligtum bei Theben. Vorläufiger bericht über die grabungskampagnen 1964–1966', *Archäologischer Anzeiger* 82, 228–273.
Burkert, W. 2001. *Greek Religion*, Oxford.
Cooper, F. and Morris, S. 1990. 'Dining in round buildings', in Murray, O. (ed.), *Sympotica: A Symposium on the Symposion*, Oxford, 66–85.
Daumas, M. 2003. 'The sanctuary of the Cabeiri', in Athanassopoulou, A. and Tzedakis, Y. (eds.), *The Bull in the Mediterranean World: Myth and Cults*, Athens, 138–143.
Dittenberger, W. 1892. *Inscriptiones Graecae VII. Inscriptiones Megaridis et Boeotiae*, Berlin.
Evans, N.A. 2002. 'Sanctuaries, sacrifices and the Eleusinian Mysteries', *Numen* 49, 227–254.
Gilhus, I.S. 2006. *Animals, Gods and Humans: Changing Attitudes to Animals in Greek, Roman and early Christian Ideas*, London.
Hamilakis, Y. 2003. 'The sacred geography of hunting: wild animals, social power and gender in early farming societies', in Kotjabopoulou, E., Hamilakis, Y., Halstead, P., Gamble, C. and Elefanti, V. (eds.), *Zooarchaeology in Greece*, London, 239–247.
Hemberg, B. 1950. *Die Kabiren*, Uppsala.
Heyder, W. and Mallwitz, A. 1978. *Die Bauten im Kabirenheiligtum bei Theben*, Berlin.
Lehmann, K. 1998. *Samothrace. A Guide to the Excavations and the Museum*, (6th edition), Thessaloniki.
Lembesi, A. 1993. 'Ta metallina zodia tou Thebaikou Kabirou: mia ermineutiki protasi', *Archaiologike Ephemeris* 131, 1–19.
Parlama, L. and Stampolidis, N.C. 2000. *Athens: The City beneath the City. Antiquities from the Metropolitan Railway Excavations*, Athens.
Reese, D.S. 1989. 'Faunal remains from the altar of Aphrodite Ourania, Athens', *Hesperia* 58, 63–70.
Reese, D.S. 2005. 'Faunal remains from Greek sanctuaries: a survey', in Hägg, R. and Alroth, B. (eds.), *Greek Sacrificial Ritual, Olympian and Chthonian. Proceedings of the Sixth International Seminar on Ancient Greek Cult*, Stockholm, 121–123.
Schachter, A. 1986. *Cults of Boiotia. II. Herakles to Poseidon*, London.
Schachter, A. 2003. 'Evolutions of a mystery cult: the Theban Kabeirion', in Cosmopoulos, M.B. (ed.), *Greek Mysteries: The Archaeology and Ritual of Ancient Greek Secret Cults*, London, 112–142.
Schmaltz, B. 1974. *Terrakotten aus dem Kabirenheiligtum bei Theben*, Berlin.
Schmaltz, B. 1980. *Metallfiguren aus dem Kabirenheiligtum bei Theben*, Berlin.
Symons, M. 2002. 'Cutting up cultures', *Journal of Historical Sociology* 15, 431–450.
Van Straten, F.T. 1995. *Hierà Kalá: Images of Animal Sacrifice in Archaic and Classical Greece*, Leiden.
Wolters, P. 1887. 'Miscellen', *Mitteilungen des Deutschen Arch. Instituts, Athenische Abteilung* 12, 269–274.
Wolters, P. 1890a. 'Das Kabirenheiligtum bei Theben. IV. Terrakotten', *Mitteilungen des Deutschen Arch. Instituts, Athenische Abteilung* 15, 355–367.
Wolters, P. 1890b. 'Das Kabirenheiligtum bei Theben. VI. Verscheidenes', *Mitteilungen des Deutschen Archäologischen Instituts, Athenische Abteilung* 15, 375–377.
Wolters, P. and Bruns, G. 1940. *Das Kabirenheiligtum bei Theben*, Berlin.

Splitting Hares! Investigating Anthropogenic Modification Signatures on Leporid Bones, using Actualistic Experiments to Improve Identifying Small Mammal Exploitation by Humans

Wendy Howard
University of Exeter

The remains of small mammals (used here to describe mesofauna the size of badger and rabbit, though not mouse-sized micromammals) are often found in archaeological deposits, but can present a problem for archaeologists. First, there are recovery issues associated with retrieving small bones, which necessitates sieving spoil with fine screens to recover a representative sample (Payne 1972; Shaffer 1982; Shaffer and Sanchez 1994), or combining water separation and soil-flotation techniques (Struever 1968, 362), all with corresponding time and workforce implications. Even when these bones are recovered, the biggest problem is identifying when they arrived in deposits as the result of human activity (Higgins 1999) rather than from natural or biological agencies, such as geological factors like soil or water action, or non-human predators (Behrensmeyer 1982; Isaac 1983; Schiffer 1987; Waters and Kuehn 1996). As with larger mammals, identifying anthropogenic use is easier when bones exhibit clear indication of human modification, such as butchery marks (for example Andersen 1994–95; Tomé 2005) or burning (Lyman 1994), but the reduced size of small mammal bones means they are less likely to be jointed or broken for cooking, marrow or grease extraction, so such evidence is often lacking. Consequently, reports on small mammal remains from archaeological sites have sometimes been reduced to a list of species present, or employed them as a proxy to reconstruct former environments (for example McNabb 2005, 296; Price 2003), perhaps with little or no further comment. Finally, there is the issue of cultural or personal bias, which can influence which species are considered to have constituted food or deemed to have been a viable source of raw material for cultural artefacts.

The combined result of these factors has meant that small mammal remains have often been overlooked for analysis (Payne 1975) or even detailed zooarchaeological examination, with a consequent loss of information about the extent of their utilization by (or interaction with) humans, whether for diet or other reasons. However, the author considers that, despite their size, small mammals were utilized more than is often thought, making it important to identify when and how such species were exploited in order to gain a more holistic understanding of past economies and lifestyles. But to achieve this, an improved methodology is needed to identify human utilization of these species from their skeletal remains. This paper describes one approach that addresses the issue of improving such identification, using actualistic experimentation to explore the visible effects of carcase preparation and dismemberment practices on raw and cooked leporid bones.

Aims

The main experiment aim was to identify the nature and appearance of certain human-induced bone modification signatures that could arise on smaller mammal bones during the course of processing, cooking, or consumption. It also examined whether the bone condition had any bearing on the way in which they disarticulated and their susceptibility to surface modification so was conducted using raw and cooked rabbit bones and joints. The intention was to treat rabbit carcases in a similar way to that in which they could be reasonably assumed to have been treated in prehistory. The experiment also questioned whether the opposite situation could be identified, and if any bone modification signature(s) could indicate the specific cooking or processing method originally employed, which could then be applied back to archaeological assemblage material. In addition, there was an experiential element to the experiment, as it allowed the processes involved in cooking and dismembering rabbit to be experienced first-hand, enabling better understanding of the species' utilization and processing from a practical and anatomical viewpoint.

One specific question stemmed from examining fracture patterns, after an unusual type of damage was noticed on bird bones recovered from Palaeolithic cave sites like La Vache (Ariège, France). These lesions comprised what was termed 'notch and medial wrench' morphology in the ulna and distal humerus of snow ptarmigan (*Lagopus lagopus*) and the radius of snowy owl (*Nyctea scandiaca*) (Laroulandie 2005; Laroulandie et al. 2008), which resembled roughly circular depressions or fractures in the olecranon fossa region of the humerus. Experiments on modern ptarmigan identified that the mechanism producing these changes was hyperextension (over-extension) of limb joints, which occurs when the joint is bent in the opposite direction to which it normally articulates. This can happen during carcase preparation, when it is divided by jointing in readiness for cooking, or is caused by people during consumption, but ultimately causes dislocation and/or breakage. The resultant characteristic breakage patterns produced range from light squashing of the olecranon fossa, the production of a hole (with or without an attached flake) on the distal humerus, to breaking off of the entire medial aspect of the articulation (Laroulandie 2005). Further experimentation into this phenomenon on uncooked sheep forelimbs by the same author identified the production of a negative wear scar on the ulnar anconeal process, which was sometimes associated with lateral crushing of the bone. Yet this modification remained unidentified on archaeological samples of small ungulates (Laroulandie et al. 2008).

Recognizing such signatures provides a useful indicator of human utilization, so this experiment aimed to determine whether the same treatment produced similar patterns on small mammal bones and identify whether joint disarticulation, by twisting or in a linear plane, produced comparable bone modification. It was hypothesized that the results should be more pronounced in mammals, given the anatomical and morphological differences between the two taxonomic classes. While the radius and ulna in most birds is of similar length, in mammals the ulna extends beyond the radius, so hyperextension of this joint in mammals could potentially impinge more profoundly on the distal humerus, creating more marked fracture patterns than in birds.

Method outline

Rabbit was selected for the experiments due to their abundance and availability, but considered a proxy for small mammals generally. The experiment was conducted on whole cooked and uncooked rabbit carcasses, to allow for the animals potentially also being consumed raw in the past. In each case the rabbit carcasses were subjected to disarticulation of their limb joints in a linear direction or using a twisting action. All were stripped of meat after cooking (this was eaten) with the joints disarticulated, and the bones cleaned by maceration; boiling or cleaning using beetles were avoided to prevent the accidental introduction of anomalous bone signatures. Once cleaned, all long bones were examined macroscopically and microscopically, using a low-magnification stereo binocular microscope at x6.7 to x45 magnification as necessary. All were examined for their overall appearance and evidence of modification or surface changes, including cut-marks and fracture evidence, such as fracture type and damage to shaft surfaces or articular ends, with all results recorded.

Cooking method

Spit-roasting and pit-roasting (Figure 3.1a and b, and described below) were the cooking methods selected for the rabbits as they were the techniques potentially employed in prehistory.

Spit-roasting

A small, sloping-sided pit *c.*50 cm in diameter and 30 cm deep was used, which was lined with granite slabs. A fire was lit within it and left to burn for an hour until the coals were hot. The rabbits had been ventrally sliced (longitudinally) when gutted, so were tied onto non-toxic hazel spits and positioned over the fire (Figure 3.1a). They were left until considered adequately cooked, with the flesh browned, as they were to be eaten (it was considered unethical to cook them and merely discard them). When cooked, the rabbits' limb joints were subjected to hyperextension in a linear or twisting direction, to mimic disarticulation. This was either done when the meat/muscle was intact, to replicate dividing up a cooked carcass, or when partially eaten, to replicate disarticulating the limbs during consumption. In each case the method used was carefully recorded, with each category bagged individually for each animal.

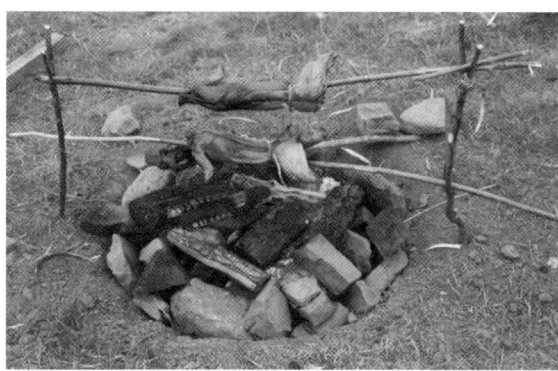

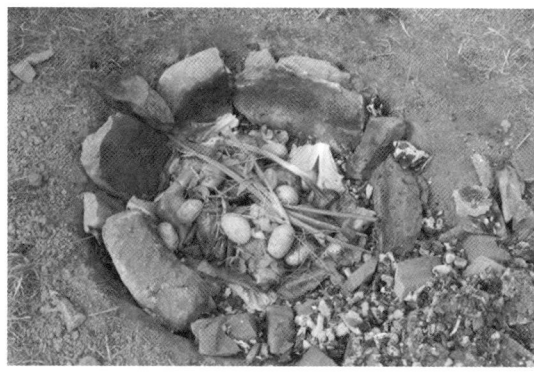

Figure 3.1. Cooking the rabbits by spit-roasting, suspending them above a pre-heated fire (top) and by pit-roasting (with vegetables) (below), using leaves to protect the meat from ash (Photos: author).

Pit roasting
When spit-roasting was completed, the ashes and hot coals were removed from the pit and a thick layer of cabbage leaves placed in it to keep the rabbits clean. The rabbits were placed on top of these with a few vegetables and herbs (Figure 3.1b), and covered with a further thick layer of leaves. The coals and hot stones were replaced quickly to minimize heat loss, and the pit covered with earth. The cooking time used was based on the time taken to spit-roast the other rabbits, plus a little extra. This slightly longer cooking time ensured the rabbits were adequately cooked for human consumption.

Experiment
Uncooked
Two rabbits were used to examine the effects of preparing fresh, uncooked carcasses for cooking. They were obtained intact with head and paws from a local butcher, already gutted but unskinned. The intention was to subject the left limb joints to linear disarticulation, and the right limbs to twisting disarticulation. However, it became

clear when trying to linearly hyperextend the elbow joints that they were simply too tough in their fleshed state, despite attempts by various individuals. This precluded the joints being torn apart by this action, and the same problem occurred when trying to disarticulate them by twisting. To resolve this, and still potentially produce some effect on the bones, the soft tissues were cut slightly and the joints then manipulated, with some tissues requiring further cutting to sever the joints completely. It is acknowledged that such action may unfortunately have severed ligaments and tendons that would have held the bones and joints in articulation, so that any manipulation following cutting may have caused the joint to disarticulate before the humerus and ulna could impinge on each other and produce fracturing or avulsion.

Cooked
The cooking component of the experiment was set up in a local field. Six rabbits were used, three each for pit-roasting and spit-roasting, all acquired from local butchers. The choice and number of rabbits used was limited by availability, but all were adults and had been shot. All had been gutted through a ventral incision and skinned prior to acquisition, with head and paws removed. Spit-roasting took 90 minutes and the pit-roasting 120 minutes, which ensured the rabbits were adequately cooked for human consumption. After cooking, the rabbits were removed from the spit and pit (and cleaned of ash for the latter), and their joints subjected to linear or twisting disarticulation. The meat was eaten, the bones recorded and bagged, and skeletonized as described above.

Results
Uncooked rabbit (Tables 3.1 and 3.2) and cooked rabbit (Tables 3.3 to 3.6)
The uncooked rabbits showed no evidence of cut-marks on bones or joint surfaces, despite cutting to sever the tough joint tendons and ligaments. No fractures were present on the articular ends of the bones, and there was no evidence of the 'notch and medial wrench' morphology seen on the birds' wing bones. Most rabbit bones remained intact during linear and twisting disarticulation of the cut joints, but in one instance twisting disarticulation resulted in a spiral fracture in the proximal shaft of an ulna, while those damaged from linear hyperextension included a scapula and ulna. The suprahamate (metacromion process) had been broken off the scapula, and there were negative 'scar and wrench' marks on the ulna of Rabbit 2 where the anconeus was damaged (Figure 3.2), with a probable area of crushing near it.

Table 3.1. Uncooked, fleshed rabbit, subjected to linear hyperextension.
(N = Normal; F = Fused; P = Proximal; D = Distal.)

	Rabbit 1 (Left limbs)		Rabbit 2 (Left limbs)	
Element	Fusion		Fusion	
Scapula	*F*	N	*F*	Fractured suprahamate
Humerus P	-	N	*PF*	N
Humerus D	-	N	*DF*	N
Ulna P	*PF*	N	*PF*	Damage to anconeus. Slightly crushed area
Ulna D	*DF*	N	*DF*	N
Radius P	*PF*	N	*PF*	N
Radius D	*DF*	N	*DF*	N
Pelvis	*F*	N	*F*	N
Femur P	*PF*	Hole on lateral side	*PF*	N
Femur D	*DF*	N	*DF*	Circular lesion on condyle
Tibia P	*PF*	N	*PF*	N
Tibia D	*DF*	N	*DF*	N

Table 3.2. Uncooked, fleshed rabbit, subjected to twisting disarticulation.
(N = Normal; F = Fused; P = Proximal; D = Distal.)

	Rabbit 1 (Right limbs)		Rabbit 2 (Right limbs)	
Element	Fusion		Fusion	
Scapula	*F*	N	*F*	N
Humerus P	-	?	*PF*	N
Humerus D	-	-	*DF*	N
Ulna P	*PF*	N	*PF*	N
Ulna D	*DF*	N	*DF*	N
Radius P	*PF*	N	*PF*	N
Radius D	*DF*	N	*DF*	N
Pelvis	*F*	N	*F*	N
Femur P	*PF*	N	*PF*	N
Femur D	*DF*	N	*DF*	Chopped
Tibia P	*PF*	N	*PF*	N
Tibia D	*DF*	N	*DF*	N

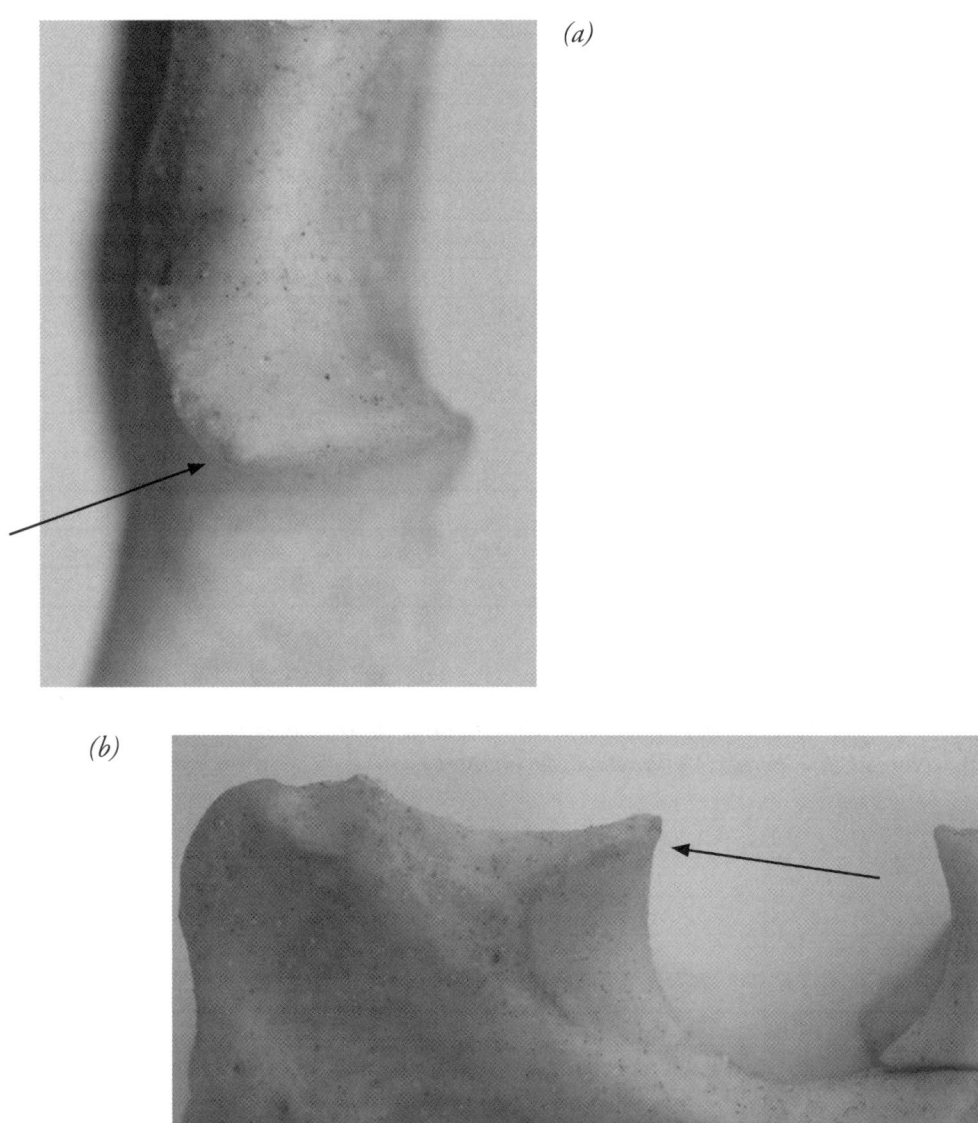

Figure 3.2. Left and below: Area chipped off the anconeus during linear hyperextension of the left elbow (arrowed). This would be caused by the trochlear of the humerus impinging on it during disarticulation (Photos: author).

Table 3.3. Spit-roasted rabbit, subjected to linear hyperextension. (N = Normal; F = Fused; P = Proximal; D = Distal;* indicates fracture related to paw removal.)

	Rabbit 1 (Left limbs)		Rabbit 2 (Left limbs)		Rabbit 3 (Right limbs)	
Element	Fusion	Meat on	Fusion	Meat off	Fusion	Meat on
Scapula		Fractured spine				Fractured spine and hamate
Humerus P	F	?Area missing?				
Humerus D	F	N		Chopped across		
Ulna P		N				Anconeus fractured
Ulna D	-	Fractured*			-	Fractured*
Radius P						
Radius D	-	Fractured*			-	Fractured*
Pelvis	F	N			F	Fractured symphysis pubis
Femur P		N		N		
Femur D		N		N		
Tibia P					-	Fractured N
Tibia D			-	Fractured*	-	Fractured*

Table 3.4. Spit-roasted rabbit, subjected to twisting disarticulation.

	Rabbit 1 (Left limbs)		Rabbit 2 (Right limbs)		Rabbit 3 (Right limbs)	
Element	Fusion	Meat on	Fusion	Meat on	Fusion	Meat off
Scapula		N		Damage to spine		Fractured inferior angle
Humerus P	NF	H	NF	Fractured during twisting	PF	N
Humerus D	F	N	F	N		N
Ulna P		N	PF	Lesion		N
Ulna D		Fractured*		Fractured*		Fractured*
Radius P		N	PF	N		N
Radius D		Fractured*		Fractured*		Fractured*
Pelvis						
Femur P						
Femur D		?Avulsion on lateral condyle		N		
Tibia P		?Tibial tubercle		?Tibial tubercle		
Tibia D		Fractured*		Fractured*		

Table 3.5. Pit-roasted rabbit, subjected to linear hyperextension.

	Rabbit 1 (Left limbs)		Rabbit 2 (Right limbs)		Rabbit 3 (Right limbs)	
Element	Fusion	Meat on	Fusion	Meat on	Fusion	Meat off
Scapula	*F*	Fractured inferior angle	*F*	Fractured inferior angle	*F*	Fractured spine + superior angle
Humerus P	*PF*	N	*PF*	N	*PF*	N
Humerus D	*DF*	N	*DF*	Chopped Discoloured	*DF*	N
Ulna P			*PF*	N	*PF*	?Scar
Ulna D			-	Fractured*	-	Fractured*
Radius P			*PF*	N	*PF*	N
Radius D			-	Fractured*	-	Fractured*
Pelvis	*F*	N	*F*	Shot	*F*	Fractured symphysis pubis
Femur P	*PF*	N	*PF*	Crazing	*PF*	N
Femur D	*DF*	N	*DF*	Crazing	*DF*	N
Tibia P	*PF*	N	*PF*	Crazing	*PF*	Brown spotting
Tibia D	-	Fractured*	-	Fractured* Marrow browned	-	Fractured*

Table 3.6. Pit-roasted rabbit, subjected to disarticulation by twisting.

	Rabbit 1 (Left limbs)		Rabbit 2 (Right limbs)		Rabbit 3 (Left limbs)	
Element	Fusion	Meat on	Fusion	Meat on	Fusion	Meat off
Scapula				Spine damaged		N
Humerus P	*F*	?Area missing?		N	*PF*	N
Humerus D	*F*	N		Chopped across	*DF*	Crazing
Ulna P		N		Lesion	*PF*	Lesion
Ulna D		Fractured*			-	Fractured*
Radius P					*PF*	N
Radius D					-	Fractured*
Pelvis					*F*	N
Femur P		N		N	*PF*	?Lesion
Femur D		N		N	*DF*	N
Tibia P					*PF*	N
Tibia D				Fractured*	-	Fractured*

Splitting Hares!

Cut-marks and surface changes

Despite using knives (and fingers) to remove the cooked meat, no cut-mark evidence was seen on any rabbit bones. All had been cooked whole with jointing carried out afterwards, so any preparation damage would be limited to that produced during gutting, head and paw removal, and skinning. The two cooking processes and variation in positioning would have exposed the rabbit carcases to different amounts of heat, but despite this there were negligible visible surface changes to any bones, with no heavy charring or significant discoloration, regardless of cooking method.

For the spit-cooked rabbit bones, the only visible colour change consisted of small localized, darkened flecks on the tip of one exposed distal tibia. Even the atlas and axis vertebrae on one spit-roasted rabbit, which had seemed browned or even slightly burned when cooking, showed no colour change following defleshing. Minute localized discoloured patches were present on two pit-roasted bones (Figure 3.3a), suggesting that the thick cabbage leaf layer protected the rabbit from direct contact with hot stones and ashes (though the bones may not have changed colour even without this). Where bones exhibited small patches of colour change it was attributed to ashes permeating down between the protective layers of leaves and singeing them. However, increased crazing (Figure 3.3b) was noticed on the humeral head of one pit-roasted rabbit, and attributed to more intense heat from its proximity to the fire and/or hot granite slabs.

Fracture damage

A number of fractures were present on cooked bones. The main ones included the distal tibiae, radii, and ulnae, and were produced by paw removal soon after killing, leaving 'fresh', helical shaft fractures. In addition, one spit-roasted rabbit sustained a spiral fracture to a humerus during twisting disarticulation. Small-scale damage was present on four pit-roasted rabbit scapulae; three of these had been disarticulated by twisting (Figure 3c), while another was damaged during linear manipulation. The resultant damage occurred at the inferior angle of two scapulae subjected to linear disarticulation, and affected the body-spine junction of the scapula in others, causing breakage to the acromion process of one, and with the suprahamate completely broken off yet another.

As with the uncooked rabbit, the most significant modification was again on a proximal ulna, where there was damage to the ulnar anconeus of one spit-roasted rabbit subjected to linear hyperextension when fully fleshed; there was also a smaller lesion on a second ulna. It appeared that a small sliver of the anconeal process had been sheared off during twisting disarticulation and was attributed to the humeral trochlea impinging on it, though avulsion of soft tissue attachments may also have contributed to the lesion. In terms of improving identification of anthropogenically modified small mammal bones the occurrence of the bone spall or fracture on the ulnar anconeal process (Figure 3.2) appears to be of most use. While this experiment produced relatively few lesions, subsequent analysis of leporid bones from two North American archaeological

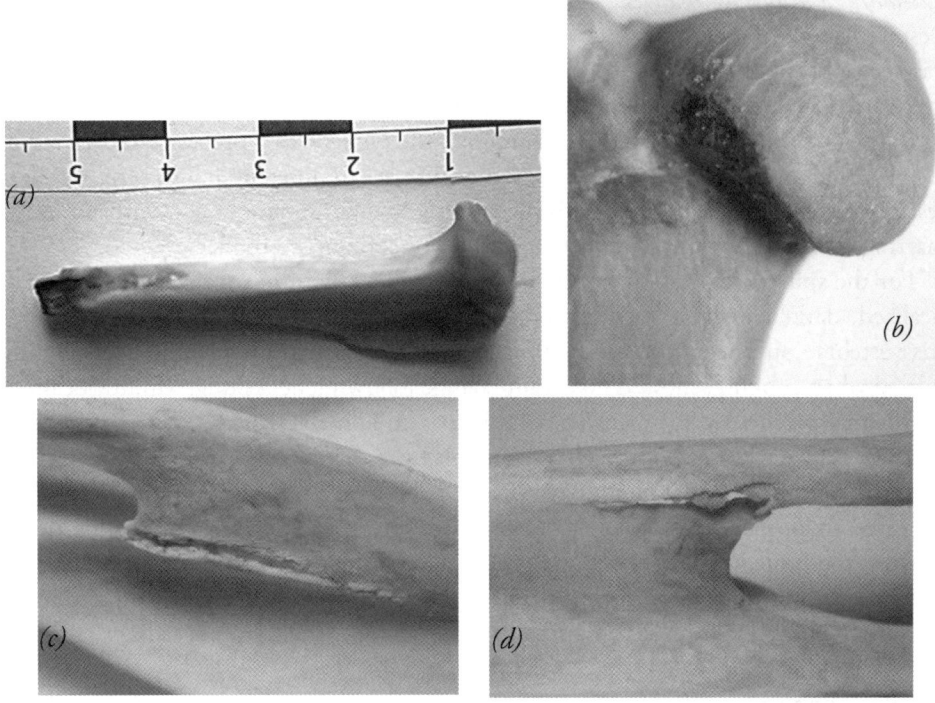

Figure 3.3. a) Burning discoloration on a distal tibia; b) Crazing on the humeral head of a pit-roasted rabbit; c and d) Breaks at the spine/body junction of spit-roasted rabbit scapulae, attributed to forelimb disarticulation (Photos: author).

sites showed it occurred quite regularly, while comparison with two 'natural' control assemblages showed no evidence of such modification (Figure 3.4).

Variations of the same lesion was identified on several ulnae subjected to linear and twisting disarticulation, but in this experiment it appeared more pronounced in cooked rabbit. As with the uncooked rabbits, there were no obvious fractures or gross damage present on any long-bone articular ends comparable to that seen on birds, nor was there other marked evidence of 'notch and medial wrench' morphology on distal humeri.

Discussion

The experiments produced relatively little bone modification or changes, despite the processes to which they were subjected. The main modifications (mostly occurring in the forelimb) are now examined with respect to colour change, cut-marks, and evidence for disarticulation and fractures.

The small degree of colour change on cooked bones is attributed to them being mainly well-covered with flesh, though more discoloration was expected on the

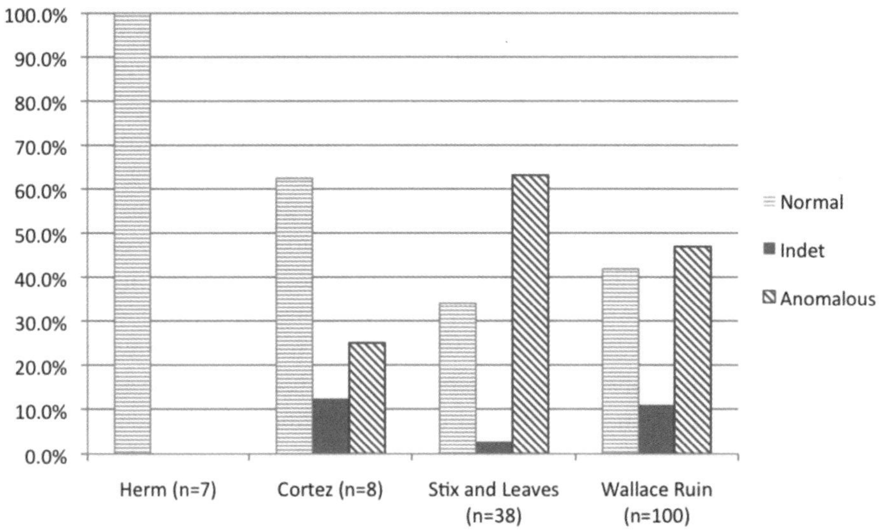

Figure 3.4: The relative frequency of damage to the proximal ulnae of leporids from two control assemblages (from Herm (Britain) and Cortez (North America)), and from two archaeological sites: Stix and Leaves pithouse (n = 38), and Wallace Ruin kiva (n = 100) (Colorado, North America).

spit-cooked rabbits given the exposed leg and neck ends during cooking and the apparent surface darkening on them at this time. Such changes could have been more pronounced had the bones protruded further beyond the flesh and more exposed to intense heat or flames. It is possible that in the past rabbits (and other small species) were cooked directly on hot coals, and this method could result in more marked colour change, even burning, to exposed bones in direct contact with heat/fire; making this a potential avenue for further experimentation. In either case it suggests that blackened, white, or calcined rabbit bones recovered from deposits must have been subjected to more intense heat or for a longer time, whether during cooking (when only part of the bone is usually affected) or following their discard into fire (the most likely scenario when the whole bone is involved).

Cooking time is a variable factor, so when considering this data relative to archaeological rabbit bones and comparing it with past utilization and treatment it must be remembered that these experiments were performed under modern controlled and timed conditions, with the criteria of what constitutes 'cooked' based on our cultural biases and preferences. The experiment rabbits were specifically cooked for enough time (two hours maximum) to make them palatable, but the treatment of such foods by other cultures could vary. Rabbits, as with any species, may have been eaten raw (even perhaps fermented), well-cooked, or somewhere in between. Prehistoric rabbits and other small mammals could have been left cooking slowly in coals, on a spit, or in a pit throughout the day, to be eaten when needed. Cooking may have been diligently observed by any member of the group or by a designated 'cook', or left unattended while people were engaged in other activities. All are factors that could affect the degree of colour change in bones, especially when their exposure to fire is significantly increased.

The general lack of cut-marks on uncooked bones is unsurprising, given that the rabbits were whole and most cutting had been through the articulations when jointing, with little knife-bone contact. Consequently, preparation damage would be limited to that caused during skinning, head and paw removal, and gutting. In addition, much meat had been removed manually, again reducing the likelihood of cut-marks. The cooked rabbits were also whole, with jointing carried out afterwards. But even examination of cooked rabbit bones where knives were used to remove meat revealed no obvious evidence of cut-marks. Different cooking methods could potentially affect the susceptibility of bone surfaces to knife damage, while more pronounced knife or lithic tool use for preparation or eating could increase the likelihood of this being present. In both cases the lack of cut-marks may simply reflect careful, unhurried meat removal by individuals, perhaps due to their unfamiliarity with eating rabbit, whereas someone who regularly ate them might have been faster and less cautious, maybe even applying a little more force.

The small degree of bone modification and fractures present was surprising given the forced linear or twisting disarticulation applied to the forelimb joints, with cooking seemingly having little effect on the bones' susceptibility to damage. Scapulae seemed the elements most susceptible to fracture damage during the experiments, which is no doubt related to their thin nature. But while damage to them might have arisen when the shoulder joints were hyperextended and the humerus impinged on the acromion process, most that were damaged were from pit-roasted rabbits. Consequently, it is possible that in some instances the weight of overlying coals and ash could have caused, or at least contributed to, such changes.

Contrary to the elbow disarticulation hypothesis, there was no pronounced evidence of 'notch and medial wrench' morphology on any forelimb bones comparable to the bird wing fractures, despite the difference in the relative lengths of the leporid radius and ulna. There are several possible explanations for this, the most likely deriving from the anatomical and physiological variation between taxa. Firstly, there are differences in the internal structure of bird and mammal bones due to the intrinsic adaptation of bird bones for flight. Mammal bones generally contain more compact bone in their long-bone shafts, so are usually more solid than the bones of many bird species which tend to be more hollow, though there is inter-species variation in bird bone structure, dependent upon whether they are predominantly adapted for flight, swimming, diving (with denser bones) or flightless (Habib and Ruff 2008). Mammal long bones also contain marrow, whereas relatively few bird long bones are marrow-bearing, again influencing the susceptibility to fractures, or the resultant type. Secondly, different forms of movement inflict different strains on joints. Bird flight tends to involve a more, rotational shoulder and elbow movement (Brown 1963; Tobalske 2007, 3139), while the cursorial and jumping movement of leporids is linear; with each producing a concomitant strain on the associated joints and muscles. Consequently the locomotory evolution of these different taxa would have resulted in the necessary anatomical modification, which could predispose bird elbows to fracture when moved in a certain plane, with those of rabbits perhaps more prone to dislocate. Finally, the lack of damage to the distal articular end of the humerus may also have been affected by the presence of the humeral aperture (the hole above the trochlea), a normal feature for *Oryctolagus cuniculus*, but occurring in a similar position to the damage site on the olecranon fossa in birds. Rabbit was selected for this experiment due to its relative ease of availability, but it would be interesting to see whether the same results were obtained from species lacking the humeral aperture morphology.

However, Cochard et al. (2012, 42) record seeing fracture patterns on leporid bones from Les Canalettes (France), a Mousterian rock-shelter, which they considered to be comparable to those on birds, and therefore the result of human activity. They report that 'the olecranon region of the ulna is generally broken (22/32 or 67.8%)… with instances of breakage near the radial fossa region of the distal humerus (4/28 or 14.3%), and may attest to the overextension of the elbow during disarticulation.' No such results were obtained from these experiments, though a larger sample size could provide a better representation of the range of fractures produced. It is possible that the bones were fresher when disarticulated, perhaps making damage more likely. Another possibility is that they were inflicted on the elbows of uncooked rabbits by stronger individuals than those attempting it for this experiment.

Conclusion

Overall, there was little colour change on any bones, despite the fact that exposed bone ends or shafts often appeared discoloured during cooking. The few changes present included dark specks on pit-roasted rabbit bones, attributed to ash, and blackened tips to fractured bone ends, though these were minimal. The same was true of cut-marks, with little evidence of this present, though bone shafts are often broken to remove paws or deliberately broken to remove marrow. Such fractures produced on the distal humerus, radius, ulna, and tibia from paw removal are useful indictors of human utilization, but the majority of bone modification produced on rabbits will inevitably be more subtle than this.

This subtlety of anthropogenic modification evidence extends to the effects of joint hyperextension, with the most significant result from this being the damage identified on the ulnar anconeal process, which may prove to be a useful method of identifying human utilization with more research. Only a small sample was examined here, and so a more statistically viable larger sample would be beneficial, as would further experimentation to confirm this as a viable means of identifying human utilization of small mammals.

While at first glance the paucity of findings may seem like a poor return, these experiments have undoubtedly been useful. Reporting the 'negative' results from the experiment, such as the minimal colour change and lack of cut-marks from the processes employed, clearly demonstrates that it is not enough to rely solely on butchery marks or burning on bones to identify anthropogenic utilization of small mammals, as utilization can evidently occur without leaving these signatures. It positively confirms the general lack of highly visible bone modification produced from significant traumatic insult to rabbits' joints when raw and cooked, and there is no obvious evidence that cooking significantly reduces or increases the likelihood of potential damage to bones, though repeating the experiment using a larger sample could prove otherwise. Finally, this experiment indicates useful areas for future work; such as using different cooking methods, cooking directly on hot coals (with whole skinned and unskinned carcases), experimenting with increasing cooking times or with varying temperatures.

Most previous research has examined anthropogenic effects on bones of larger mammals, rather than smaller ones, and this work is a positive step towards disproving some of the assumptions about the changes to leporid bones that result from activities like carcase processing and cooking. What these experiments clearly show is the lack of changes produced on raw and cooked bones despite different disarticulation and cooking methods, with this work disproving some conjecture about bone changes from such treatment and the nature of those modifications. There have been, and still are, a lot of assumptions about how smaller species were used as a dietary resource, both in terms of the species actually utilized, acquisition techniques, the ways in which they were prepared and cooked, and the type of bone modification signatures resulting from such action. Little work has been done to confirm or refute many of these assumptions, and this paper goes some small way towards addressing this.

Acknowledgements

I am particularly grateful to Alan Outram for his advice and comments on aspects of this experiment, and for supervising my PhD thesis from which this study arose. This experiment was part of my doctoral research funded by the Arts and Humanities Research Council. I am very grateful to Catherine Norman and Benny Venn for allowing me to carry out these experiments in their field, and to members of ACE Archaeology Club (Mid-Devon) for their assistance. Thanks also to Peter Leeming for remarks made on an earlier draft of this paper, and to the anonymous reviewer for their useful comments. Any mistakes that remain, however, are entirely my own.

References

Andersen, S.H. 1994–95. 'Ringkloster Ertebolle trappers and wild boar hunters in eastern Jutland: A survey', *Journal of Danish Archaeology* 12, 13–59.

Behrensmeyer, A.K. 1982. 'Time resolution in fluvial vertebrate assemblages', *Paleobiology* 8(3), 211–227.

Brown, R.H.J. 1963. 'The flight of birds', *Biological Reviews* 38(4), 460–489.

Cochard, D., Brugal, J.-P., Morin, E. and Meignen, L. 2012. 'Evidence of small fast game exploitation in the Middle Paleolithic of Les Canalettes Aveyron, France', *Quaternary International* 264, 32–51.

Habib, M.B. and Ruff, C.B. 2008. 'The effects of locomotion on the structural characteristics of avian limb bones', *Zoological Journal of the Linnean Society* 153(3), 601–624.

Higgins, J. 1999. 'Túnel: A Case Study of Avian Zooarchaeology and Taphonomy', *Journal of Archaeological Science* 26(12), 1449–1457.

Isaac, G. 1983. 'Bones in Contention: Competing Explanations for the Juxtaposition of Early Pleistocene Artifacts and Faunal Remains', in Clutton-Brock, J. and Grigson, C. (eds.), *Animals and Archaeology: 1. Hunters and their Prey*, B.A.R. International Series 163, Oxford, 3–19.

Laroulandie, V. 2005. 'Bird exploitation pattern: the case of Ptarmigan *Lagopus* sp. in the Upper Magdalenian site of La Vache (Ariège, France)', in Grupe, G. and Peters, J. (eds.), *Feathers, Grit and Symbolism. Birds and Humans in the Ancient Old and New Worlds. Proceedings of the 5th Meeting of the ICAZ Bird Working Group, Munich, 26–28 July 2004*, Documenta Archaeobiologiae 3, 165–178.

Laroulandie, V., Costamagno, S., Cochard, D., Mallye, J.-B., Beauval, C., Castel, J.-C., Ferrié, J.-G., Gourichon, L. and Rendu, W. 2008. 'Quand désarticuler laisse des traces: le cas de l'hyperextension du coude', *Annals de Paléontologie* 94, 287–302.

Lyman, R.L. 1994. *Vertebrate Taphonomy*, Cambridge.

McNabb, J. 2005. 'Hominins and the Early-Middle Pleistocene Transition: Evolution, culture and climate in Africa and Europe', in Head, M.J. and Gibbard, P.L. (eds.), *Early-Middle Pleistocene Transitions: The Land-ocean Evidence*, London, 287–304.

Payne, S. 1972. 'Partial Recovery and Sample Bias: the Results of some Sieving Experiments', in Higgs, E.S. (ed.), *Papers in Economic Prehistory*, Cambridge, 49–64.

Payne, S. 1975. 'Partial recovery and sample bias', in Clason, A.T. (ed.), *Archaeozoological Studies*, Amsterdam, 7–17.

Price, C.R. 2003. *Late Pleistocene and Early Holocene Small Mammals in South West Britain*. BAR International Series 347, Oxford.

Schiffer, M. 1987. *Formation Processes of the Archaeological Record*, Albuquerque.

Shaffer, B.S. 1992. 'Quarter-Inch Screening: Understanding Biases in Recovery of Vertebrate Faunal Remains', *American Antiquity* 57(1), 129–136.

Shaffer, B.S. and Sanchez, J.L.J. 1994. 'Comparison of ⅛'- and ¼'-mesh recovery of controlled samples of small-to-medium-sized mammals', *American Antiquity* 59(3), 525–530.

Struever, S. 1968. 'Flotation Techniques for the Recovery of Small-Scale Archaeological Remains', *American Antiquity* 33(3), 353–362.

Tobalske, B.W. 2007. 'Biomechanics of bird flight', *The Journal of Experimental Biology* 210, 3135–3146.

Tomé, C. 2005. 'Les Marmottes de la grotte Colomb (Vercors – France)', *Revue de Paléobiologie, Genève* 10, 11–21.

Waters, M.R. and Kuehn, D.D. 1996. 'The Geoarchaeology of Place: The Effect of Geological Processes on the Preservation and Interpretation of the Archaeological Record', *American Antiquity* 61(3), 483–497.

Honey Hunting, Beekeeping and the Uses and Role of Bee Products in British Prehistory

Magnhild Peggy Gilje

In 1951 Fraser wrote that: 'We can only speculate about the progress of beekeeping between Neolithic times and the dawn of written history when bees were already kept in hives of a fixed pattern and in accordance with a well-established system.' (Fraser 1951, 1). Today one could argue that further research using modern methods could shed more light on the use of bees and bee products in British prehistory. *Apis mellifera* the species of honeybee relevant to this study came to Britain following the spread of thermophile deciduous species such as lime and hazel, which only became possible in the warm post glacial period 8000–10000 years BP (Ruttner 1988, 35). It is clear that honey and wax were used in prehistory; what remains unclear is to what extent honeybees were exploited, how this was accomplished, and what importance honey and other bee products could have had in British prehistory.

Bee products

Honey, as well as being highly calorific with 64 calories per tablespoon (Khan et al. 2007, 1705), has long been used as a remedy for both internal and external ailments. For example, honey is the main ingredient in an Egyptian prescription for a wound salve discovered in the Smith Papyrus dated to 2600–2200BC (Zuma and Lulat 1989, 389). Recently honey has been used to help treat many disorders including: abrasions, amputations, bed sores, burst abdominal wounds, cervical ulcers, cracked nipples, foot ulcers in diabetics and lepers, large septic wounds, ulcers of many different types and surgical wounds both internal and external (Zumla 1989; Molan 2001; Gollu et al. 2008). Apart from honey the main contribution bee products can make to diet is bee brood, edible bee larvae. This is a much enjoyed food type in many parts of the world, including Japan (where you can buy it tinned) and many African countries (Crane 1990, 468).

Wax is another bee product, which due to its constant and impermeable properties has been used to waterproof textiles, basketry and pottery, and also as a sealant to seal lids in place on vessels. It can also be used to treat materials such as leather, wood and stone for aesthetic purposes – the wax gives a smooth glossy appearance as well as reducing wear and tear (Crane 1999, 533).

Propolis is a dark, sticky, resinous substance used by bees to seal hive walls and entrances, as well as to strengthen and reinforce borders of combs and embalm invaders that are too large to eject from the hive (Kujumgiev et al. 1999, 235). It is processed by the bees using substances secreted by plants, especially substances from wounds in the plant, liphophilic materials on leaves, leaf buds, resin, mucilage, gums and lattices (Bankova 2005, 115). All propolis has antibacterial and antifungal properties as well as most of them being antiviral (Kujumgiev et al. 1999, 239). Because of these medicinal properties propolis was frequently used in traditional medicine and in the Balkan states it is still successfully used to treat wounds, burns and stomach ulcers and many other ailments (Bankova 2005, 115).

Ways of exploiting bees as a resource

There are three main categories of bee exploitation: hive beekeeping, forest beekeeping and honey hunting. The basic principal of honey hunting or gathering is to find a colony and raid it for honey, brood and wax. The earliest know archaeological evidence of this practice is a Mesolithic painting from the La Arana shelter in Bicorp, Spain, which shows a figure carrying a container whilst ascending a ladder or rope and dipping her/his hand into a nest of bees (Crane 1983, 21). There are still many societies that practice this technique and to illustrate this a few examples will be presented.

The Efe and Mbuti tribes (collectively known as the Bambuti) of the Ituri forest in the present Democratic Republic of Congo have a whole season named after honey. They move from the outskirts of the forests to the middle, and during this season up to 80% of their calorie intake can be from honey (Ichikawa 1982, 56; Terashima 1998, 123). The Ache of eastern Paraguay are also honey hunters and their diet will at some times of the year contain large quantities of honey, accounting for up to 44% of their calorie intake (Hill et al. 1984, 119). In terms of common material culture a key feature apart from rope, containers and sharp tools, such as an axe to open the nests and access the honey, is some form of smoking device. A smoking device could be anything from a soggy smoking torch to a smoking tube, as used by the Bambuti (Ichikawa 1982, 59).

Forest beekeeping may appear very similar to honey hunting but is in fact a more ownership based system. Technically forest beekeeping can involve the enlargement of holes in trees to make suitable nesting sites for bee colonies, the fitting of doors in the tree trunks, cutting steps in trees to ease access to the honey and marking nests with ownership marks (Crane 1999, 127). Forest beekeeping was practiced over much of Europe and Russia until not long ago. Indeed, a recently abandoned living tree with a door and extended nesting area was found in the New Forest in 1978 (Crane 1983, 88). This shows that although forest beekeeping is often regarded as the intermediate stage between honey hunting and hive beekeeping (Crane 1983, 77), it can in fact coexist with the latter.

Hive beekeeping is the management of a colony of bees and encouraging it to build a nest inside a container which has a flight entrance small enough for the bees to defend, and another larger opening where the beekeeper can extract honey and wax. There is a great variety of hive types ranging from upright log hives to horizontal mud hives and only a very few examples can be presented here. A hollow oak trunk excavated in Vehne-Moor (Germany) and dated to AD 400–500 is very similar to hives found both in Europe and America. Eva Crane recorded examples of upright log hives from Poland in 1960, France in 1962 and Carolina, North America in 1960, and in fact she notes that only in the 1960s and '70s did beekeepers in Germany make a serious shift from log hives (with doors) to modern hives that open at the top (Crane 1983, 98). In terms of what would generally be preserved archaeologically there are examples of log hives found in France in 1962 where large flat slates were used as log hive lids and bases (Crane 1983, 95). These slates would not only keep out damp from below but also protect from rain and predators from above. Such slates if found archaeologically would not generally be interpreted as log hive 'toppers', and it provides an interesting example of material culture that not only would be hard to recognize but that could also have had many other uses in their lifetime. There are many examples of horizontal hives and in fact it seems that the earliest identified hives are of this type. At the Iron Age city site of Tel Rehov in the Jordan Valley eight cylinders were found aligned north to south on a wooden beam. The identification of the cylinders as hives was based on pictorial, literary and ethnographic analogies as well as residue analysis confirming the presence of wax (Mazar et al. 2008, 631). In Greece and the Aegean Islands hives have been excavated that are very similar to hives used in traditional beekeeping in the area. A paper written by Bikos and Rammou is a summary of a survey carried out of traditional beehives used on Aegean Islands conducted since 1993, aiming to be a comparative tool that can be used to better understand archaeological finds (Bikos and Rammou 2002, 6).

Eva Crane suggests that keeping bees in skeps, containers made from reeds, grasses or flexible twigs, would have been possible well before log hives were used and could in fact have been one of the first types of hive to be used together with sun-dried mud hives (Crane 1983, 99). Unfortunately there is no archaeological evidence (that I know of) to support this theory. The earliest known archaeological example dates to AD 1–200 and was excavated in the 1970s from a bog in Wierde in Germany, and both illustrations and descriptions suggest it is very similar to later medieval examples and indeed similar to skeps used until quite recently in Britain (Crane 1983, 100). The technology to make skeps was certainly available from very early on, as evidenced by the Mesolithic site of Noyen-sur-Seine in France where several remains of basketry were excavated as well six examples of intricate and delicately woven fish traps (Mordant and Mordant 1992, 61).

Due to the material that skeps are made from they are prone to rot in wet conditions. Over time this problem has been solved in a number of ways. Skeps were placed on four post wooden bench structures, wicker skeps were covered in dung and clay and the more weatherproof straw skeps were covered to prevent rain getting in. The covers could be made of thatch or anything else convenient that came to hand (Mace 1952, 16–18). A particularly interesting common factor is that most of the hives described here can be (and often are) put on simple four post structures to keep the bees off the damp ground, and so keep to a minimum attacks by such pests as ants and mice as well as deter rot. These structures would archaeologically only be visible as four postholes – something which in Britain certainly would not immediately be interpreted as a structure for the elevation of beehives.

Eva Crane suggests that hive beekeeping developed as a result of one or more of the following factors; increase in bee populations coupled with a lack of natural nesting sites, an increased need for honey and wax due to increasing human populations, and sedentary populations practicing agriculture and perhaps leaving items lying around that would be suitable for a colony to nest in (Crane 1999, 161). Unfortunately, from an archaeological point of view bees do not change physically when they are exploited by humans, they do not effectively become 'domestic' (Ruttner 1988) and cannot therefore be recognized as such in the archaeological record.

Archaeological evidence from Britain

Most of the clear evidence of the presence of bees comes in the form of entomological remains and residue of beeswax in vessels. Excavations at the site at Runnymede Bridge, discovered in 1978, recovered a large amount of Bronze Age evidence and extensive Neolithic remains, which had benefitted from being waterlogged (Needham and Evans 1987, 21). Twenty-two sherds from the waterlogged levels and which had charred material on them were selected and sent for analysis with gas-liquid chromatography (GLC) and high performance liquid chromatography (HPLC). Thirteen of the sherds were too highly carbonized to be of any use but the remaining seven sherds yielded positive results and showed the presence of beeswax on one sherd (Needham et al. 1987, 22–25). The remains of a honeybee were also found in the Bronze Age levels at the excavations at Runnymede Bridge (Robinson 2000, 146).

An example of further residue analysis is a three-part study by Copley and Evershed called *Dairying in Antiquity*, which discussed evidence from absorbed lipid residues in pottery. The study included evidence from four Iron Age sites (Copley et al. 2005a, 486), four Bronze Age sites (Copley et al. 2005b, 505) and five Neolithic sites (Copley et al. 2005c, 523). A total of 931 sherds were examined, the selected sherds from each site were rim and body sherds from vessels thought to have been used for cooking. The study found that some sherds from all three periods contained beeswax (Copley et al. 2005a, b, c). Copley et al. acknowledge that it is possible that other types of vessel may produce even more positive results in terms of beeswax and suggest lamps and combed wares as possible items for study as these have been proved useful in other parts of Europe.

During the excavation of four Bronze Ages cist burials in Ashgrove, Fife it was discovered that unusual amounts of macrobotanical remains were preserved in one of them (Dickson 1978, 108). Pollen analysis was also carried out on samples from the grave itself and the beaker vessel from within the grave. The samples showed remarkably high proportions of lime (*Tilia cordata*) pollen which was not indigenous to Scotland, as indeed it still is not. It is thought that the high quantities of lime pollen and presence of meadow sweet (*Filpendula ulmaria*) pollen indicates the presence of mead, as honey could have been transported from further south in Britain where lime was growing (Dickson 1978, 109–111).

These case studies demonstrate that there is some evidence of the use of bee products in British prehistory. What is greatly lacking is any firm knowledge of what type of exploitation took place and on what scale. There is a great void of knowledge in the area and there are several avenues of study that need to be pursued.

Further studies

It would be reasonable to assume that the careful study of ethnographic evidence could help us understand the material culture associated with beekeeping and the use of bee products we could be looking for in a British context. In terms of evidence for hives what should be sought after in the archaeological record are containers of a suitable size (in the wild *A. mellifera* will generally choose cavities no small than ten litres and no greater than one hundred litres (Akratankul 1990, 1D), with a flight entrance. So far I do not know of any such vessels that can be convincingly argued to be hives, but perhaps with further examinations of excavation reports and new excavations, some such containers will be discovered in the British Isles. The biggest problem that we face is that many of the containers seen in ethnographic evidence are made of organic materials that only survive archaeologically in very unusual circumstances. Those hives that are not of organic materials are mainly pottery and stone and found around the Mediterranean and Middle East and it would be useful to conduct experimental studies determining what type of beehives would be viable in the British Isles in 10,000 BP. Would for example pottery hives be as useful in this climate as in the Mediterranean one?

What is most needed in terms of residue analysis is a highly systematic study similar to that of *Dairying in Antiquity* (Copley et al. 2005). The study should be conducted with bee products in mind and instead of cookery vessels being sampled, pygmy vessels suitable for lamps, beakers and perforated vessels and perhaps other types of vessels yet to be indentified as significant should be examined. Another aspect of residue analysis that could be explored is that of pollen. If a pattern of pollen presence in honey, i.e. a signature of pollens that would not otherwise be found together could be determined, this could identify a container that has been used to hold bee products. Though this may be somewhat difficult, as bees would forage in similar areas to the people who exploited them, perhaps say if the pollen of plants that are toxic to humans, but useful to bees were found in cookery vessels this could indicate presence of honey.

Lost wax moulds should also be studied further to understand the scale of wax use. Lost wax casting uses wax, as the name suggests, and it has also been suggested that open stone moulds characteristic of the Bronze Age were in fact not intended as a cast for the bronze itself but for the wax models later to be used for lost wax casting (Underwood 1958; Clarke 1942, 212).

The potential for entomological evidence could be high if research was done into the significance of bee distribution on a site, answering such questions as: Where do bees die? What do bees in the colony do with their dead? How many bees on average die in or near the colony and how many die on foraging trips? This needs to be studied in greater depth to understand the significance of deposited bees in an archaeological context.

With regards to evidence of honey hunting and forest beekeeping the associated material culture is likely to be extremely ephemeral. What can be assessed to a certain level is how people used the landscape around them. In 2003 Conneller and Schadla-Hall explored the complexity of Mesolithic activity patterns in the Vale of Pickering. They concluded that no sites can be considered in isolation and that the landscape of the Vale of Pickering was a familiar one to those who lived within it (Conneller and Schadla-Hall 2003, 105). This familiarity in a landscape, with different seasonal settlements would form a good basis for knowing and exploiting resources such as bees, both in an opportunistic honey hunting manner, and in the more planned and calculated way of forest beekeeping. However it seems unlikely that any evidence of this would survive archaeologically and any evidence that may be found such as axes and ropes could be used for many purposes and may not necessarily be associated with apiculture in any shape or form. The study of beekeeping in British prehistory is one that is in its infancy. Whatever work that is done in the future will make a valuable contribution to the understanding of the exploitation of a most valuable resource, in terms of its use as a craft material as well as its nutritional and medicinal uses.

References

Akratanakul, P. 1990. 'Beekeeping in Asia', *Agricultural Food Services Bulletin* 68/4, 1D, Agriculture and Consumer Protection, Rome.
Bankova, V. 2005. 'Chemical diversity of Propolis and the Problem of Standardization', *Journal of Ethnopharmacology* 100, 114–117.
Bikos, T. and Rammou, E. 2002. 'Beehives of the Aegean Islands', *Bee World* 83(1), 5–13.
Clarke, J.G.D. 1942. 'Bees in Antiquity', *Antiquity* 16, 208–215.
Conneller, C. Schadla-Hall, T. 2003. 'Beyond Star Carr: The Vale of Pickering in the 10th Millennium BP.', *Proceedings of the Prehistoric Society* 69, 85–105.
Copley, M.S., Berstan, R., Budd, S.N., Straker, V., Payne, S. and Evershed, R.P. 2005a. 'Dairying in antiquity. I. Evidence from Absorbed Lipid residues dating to the British Iron Age', *Journal of Archaeological Science* 32, 485–503.
Copley, M.S., Berstan, R., Straker, V., Payne, S. and Evershed, R.P. 2005b. 'Dairying in antiquity. II. Evidence from Absorbed Lipid Residues dating to the British Bronze Age', *Journal of Archaeological Science* 32, 505–521.
Copley, M.S., Berstan, R., Mukherjee, A.J., Dudd, S.N., Straker, V., Payne, S. and Evershed, R.P. 2005c. 'Dairying in antiquity. III. Evidence from Absorbed Lipid Residues dating to the British Neolithic', *Journal of Archaeological Science* 32, 523–546.
Crane, E. 1983. *The Archaeology of Beekeeping*, London.
Crane, E. 1990. *Bees and Beekeeping, Science, Practice and World Resources*, New York.
Crane, E. 1999. *The World History of Beekeeping and Honey Hunting*, London.
Dickson, J.H. 1978. 'Bronze Age Mead', *Antiquity* 52, 108–113.
Fraser, M. 1951. *Beekeeping in Antiquity*, London.
Gollu, A., Kismet, K., Kilicoglu, B., Erel, S., Gonultas, M.A., Sunay, A.E. and Akkus, M.A. 2008. 'Effect of

Honey on Intestinal Morphology, Intra-abdominal Adhesions and Anastomotic Healing', *Phytotherapy Research* 22, 1243–1247.

Hill, K., Hawkes, K., Hurtado, M. and Source, H.K. 1984. 'Seasonal Variance in the Diet of Ache Hunter-Gatherers in Eastern Paraguay Human', *Ecology* 12(2), 101–135.

Ichikawa, M. 1982. 'Ecological and Sociological Importance of Honey to the Mbuti Net Hunters, Eastern Zaire', *African Study Monographs* 1, 55–68.

Khan, F.R., Abadin, Z.Ul. and Rauf, N. 2007. 'Honey: Nutritional and Medicinal Value', *International Journal of Clinical Practice* 61, 10, 1705–1707.

Kujumgiev, A., Tsvetkova, I., Serkedjieva, Y., Bankova, V., Christov, R. and Popov, V. 1999. 'Antibacterial, Antifungal and Antiviral Activity of Propolis of Different Geographic Origin', *Journal of Ethnopharmacology* 64, 235–240.

Mace, H. 1952. *The Beekeepers Handbook*, London.

Mazar, A., Namdar, D., Panitz-Cohen, N., Neumann, R. and Weiner, S. 2007. 'Iron Age Beehives at Tel Rehov in the Jordan Valley', *Antiquity* 82, 629–639.

Molan, P. 2001. 'Why Honey is Effective as a Medicine: Its use in Modern Medicine', in Munn, P. and Jones, R. (eds.), *Honey and Healing*, Cardiff, 5–14.

Mordant, C. and Mordant, D. 1992. 'Noyen-sur-Seine: a Mesolithic waterside settlement' in Coles, B. (ed.), *The Wetland Revolution in Prehistory*, Exeter, 55–64.

Needham, S. and Evans, J. 1987. 'Honey and Dripping: Neolithic Food Residues from Runnymede Bridge', *Oxford Journal of Archaeology* 6(1), 21–29, Oxford.

Robinson, M.A. 2000. 'Middle Mesolithic to Late Bronze Age Insect Assemblages and an Early Neolithic Assemblage of Waterlogged Macroscopic Plant Remains', in Needham, S. (ed.), *The passage of the Thames, Holocene and Environment and Settlement at Runnymede*, London, 146–167.

Ruttner, F. 1988. *Biogeography and Taxonomy of Honeybees*, Heildelberg.

Terashima, H. 1998. 'Honey and Holidays: The Interactions Mediated by Honey Between Efe Hunter-Gatherers and Lese Farmers, in the Ituri Forest', *African Study monograph* (Supplementary issue) 25, 123–134.

Underwood, L. 1958. 'Bronze Age Technology in Western Asia and Northern Europe: Part I', *Man* 58, 17–22.

Zumla, A. and Lulat, A. 1989. 'Honey–a Remedy Rediscovered', *Journal of the Royal Society of Medicine* 82, 384–385.

The Craft of the Maltster

Merryn Dineley

Malting, once known as 'the ubiquitous craft', was a common skill in the British Isles, with at least one maltster in every hamlet, village and small town. The specialized, traditional skills of the maltster and the brewer have been separate crafts for hundreds of years (Stopes 1885). The maltster processes harvested grain into malt by first steeping it, then germinating it on a smooth, level floor within a dark barn or other suitable building before finally drying it, gently and carefully, in the kiln. The brewer buys the malt and processes it into ale or beer.

Today, few people know what malt is nor how it is made. The ancient and traditional craft of floor malting has become virtually invisible in the modern world. There are just a few companies left in the British Isles that still make malt in this traditional way, by steeping, then germinating grain on the floor before kilning. This paper investigates how old the traditional craft of the maltster might be. Could the craft of malting have been discovered by the earliest agriculturalists, over ten thousand years ago? As Ivor Murrell, retired Director General of the Maltsters Association of Great Britain, writes:

> Maltsters are continually surprised by how little is known about what they do, and why they do it. Perhaps we have overplayed the 'art and mystery of malting' over the years to the extent that it has become a 'secret'? We now find that some people are beginning to think that beer is made from hops and, whilst nobody would deny the significance of hops, it does indicate that malt should reveal its true importance. Outside the industry, most people know little, if anything, about it, yet malt has a long history, and a very strong story, and it is worth telling. (Murrell 2006)

What is malt?
Malt is cereal grain in which germination has been deliberately initiated and then halted by gentle drying in a kiln (Hough 1985, 4). Any grain can be malted – barley, wheat, rye or oats – but barley is the most commonly used grain for this purpose. The maltster has the necessary and specific skills to oversee the steeping of the grain, the controlled germination, when it is spread out on the floor, and finally, the drying of malt in a kiln. Malt is dried at moderate temperatures, to avoid destroying the starch-converting enzymes unless it is to be used as a specialist malt, for colouring or flavouring the ale or beer. Malt is not fully sprouted grain. It is grain in an early stage of germination, with roots and shoot (the acrospire) being no more than two-thirds of the length of the grain.

The Craft of the Maltster

Malt and water are the main ingredients for ale and beer. When the brewer heats crushed malt with warm water in the mash tun it produces a sweet mash. A liquid, known as the wort, can be extracted by lautering, then sparging or rinsing the mash with hot water (Line 1985). Wort has a delicious, sweet, malty taste. It provides all of the necessary sugars for alcoholic fermentation into ale and beer. Today hops are used to preserve and flavour beer. These replace gruit which is a mixture of plants, for example heather, yarrow and bog myrtle, used by brewers until medieval times when hops were introduced (Kistemaker and van Vilsteren 1994, 20–28; Dineley 2004, 13–18; Hornsey 2003, 269). Herbs, plant extracts, flowers or hops are the flavouring and preservatives of ale and beer and do not provide fermentable sugars.

Grain germination physiology

In sufficiently moist and aerated conditions, the embryo of the grain releases growth hormones (gibberellins) which stimulate the production of alpha amylase in the embryo and aleurone layer (Figure 5.1). This enzyme converts grain starch into maltose and glucose, the food source for the growing plant (Hough 1985, 14). If the grain grows too much, there will be no starch left for the brewer to convert into fermentable sugars, so the malt is dried when the rootlets are about one-third the length of grain. Malt stores well, provided that it is kept in dry conditions.

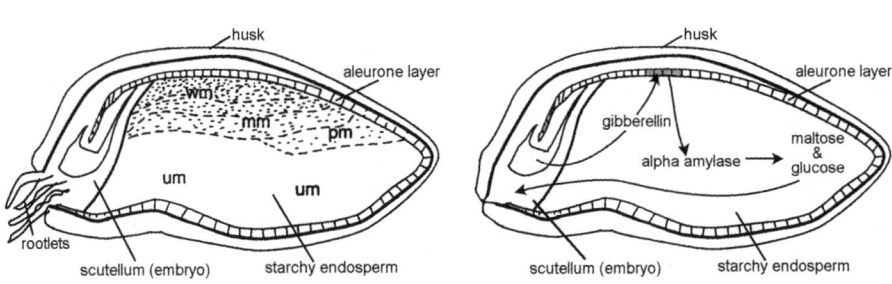

Figure 5.1. Sections through barley grain, showing the biochemical pathways of germination. Left, when grain has been steeped growth hormones (gibberellins) are activated. These stimulate the production of enzymes (amylase) from the embryo and also from the single layer of cells beneath the husk, the aleurone layer. Enzymes convert the starchy endosperm into maltose and glucose, the food source for the growing plant. Right, malt is dried in a kiln when rootlets begin to show. The malt is partially modified into maltose. The starchy endosperm is wholly modified (wm), mostly modified (mm), partially modified (pm) and unmodified (um). The husk becomes friable (after Bewley and Black 1994, 360).

The Craft of the Maltster

Malting in history and prehistory: written evidence.

The earliest written references to malt and beer are on Sumerian clay tablets dating from the Uruk period, fourth millennium BC (Hornsey 2003, 79–113). Later Sumerian documents describe how to make malt and brew beer, for example, the Hymn to Ninkasi. Dating from *c.* 1800 BC, it is a song of praise to Ninkasi, the Goddess of brewing and is a recipe or instructions for malt and ale manufacture (Civil 1964). As today, the malt was made by steeping the grain in water, then it was spread out on a floor before being dried in the sun. According to the Hymn, the malt was guarded by dogs because it was such a valuable commodity.

Floor malting techniques and traditions seem to have remained unchanged across the millennia. Descriptions of malting and brewing in Sumerian and ancient Egyptian texts closely resemble descriptions from farms, large households and monasteries in medieval and later Britain (Cobbett 1821; Firth 1922; Bennett 1996). By the sixteenth century, malting had become the most regulated agricultural activity of all. Laws were passed, stipulating a minimum of 21 days for steeping, germination and drying to ensure that good malt was always made (Stopes 1885). There is an accurate description of malting in Henry's *History of England*, published in 1770:

> Grain is steeped and germinated, by which its' spirits are excited and set free; it is then dried and ground and infused in water, when, after fermentation, it produces a pleasant, warming, strengthening and intoxicating liquor. (Stopes 1885, 5)

It is clear that, for a long time, maltsters have been able to make good quality malt without needing to understand the biochemistry of grain germination physiology. The processes of steeping, partial germination and drying can be seen as rituals, with specific conditions necessary for the success of each stage. One example of this specialist knowledge is the 'maltster's rub', whereby the maltster decides how the modification of the grain on the floors is progressing:

> a single grain is guillotined in half, between the thumb and forefinger, half the corn is discarded and the starch squeezed out of the grain husk, again between thumb and forefinger. As soon as the starch is clear of the husk, the husk is dropped, and the starch rolled between thumb and forefinger. If it smooths out like damp flour, it is ready for the kiln, if it rolls in a ball, the starch walls have not fully degraded and more flooring time is needed. (Murrell, pers. comm. 2010)

Until the eighteenth century, most farmers and rural householders knew how to make their own malt from their barley. In *Cottage Economy*, first published in 1821, Cobbett observes that, 40 years previously, to have a house or a farm and not know how to make malt and brew beer was a rare thing. There was not a labourer in the Parish, he claims, that did not make his own malt and brew his own beer. By the early nineteenth century, he despairs that 'there is not one who does it, except by chance the malt be given to him' (Cobbett 1821, 13). It was around this time that malting became a large-scale industrial process, based in the towns, often beside canals. The advent of improved transport meant that grain could be transported quickly from the field to the industrial malt house and then to the brewery. So the need for small, local maltings declined and maltings became huge industrial buildings (Figure 5.2).

Malting in prehistory: archaeological evidence

The steep
There is little evidence for this part of the process because minimal equipment is needed. Traditionally, grain is put into a porous bag to steep in a shallow stream, thus providing the necessary water and oxygen. A large vessel can be used for steeping. The water must be changed regularly and the grain given air rests. If grain is left too long in the water it will spoil. Correctly steeping the grain, in preparation for floor malting, requires skill and experience.

The malting floor
A malting floor is a smooth surface in a dark, well-ventilated building upon which the germinating grain is spread, protected from birds, beasts and the elements. The malt is turned regularly to prevent excess root growth and to allow the excess heat of germination to escape (Murrell, pers. comm.). A malting floor can be made of beaten earth, clay, wood or stone. It must be well-maintained to avoid losing malt in the cracks (Firth 1922).

A feature of some of the buildings of the early agricultural settlements in the Fertile Crescent is a well-made floor, carefully constructed and often repaired, made of beaten earth, clay or lime plaster and located in a mud brick building. Hearths, quern stones and ovens are often found in association with these floors, indicating grain processing activity, possibly malting. The function of these well-made floors is rarely discussed in excavation reports. Floors are for walking upon, for dancing, perhaps, or just for daily living. Malting should be considered as a possible function. A smooth, level, well-maintained floor within a dark but well-ventilated building is an essential requirement for the maltster.

At Ain Mallaha, a Natufian village *c.* 10,000–8200 BC, deliberately made, well-maintained floors were excavated (Maisels 1990). They were described as having been made by accumulation. There were several layers, indicating regular maintenance and repair. Floors made of compacted red clay were found at Mureybit, 8500–6900 BC, a settlement beside the Euphrates River in Syria (van Loon 1968). There were associated sickles, pestles, mortars, quern stones, fire pits and hearths (Maisels 1990, 85–86). This building may have been suitable for making malt and processing it into malt sugars.

The Craft of the Maltster

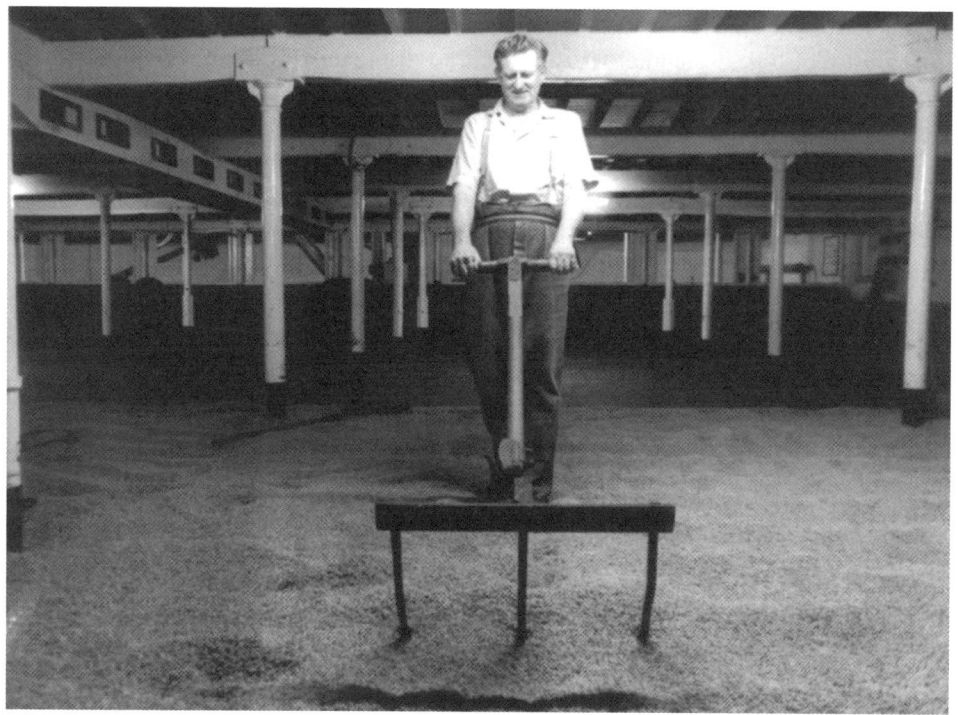

Figure 5.2: Turning the malt at Bury Maltings with a duck foot rake. The photo shows only a small area of the malting floor in use. The cleared floor area behind is waiting for the next steep to be emptied on it. (Photo: copyright Ivor Murrrell).

Stamped mud floors, surfaced with a layer of clay, were found at Ali Kosh, *c.* 7000 BC, a village in the southern plains of Khuzistan (Maisels 1990, 101).

At Beidha (*c.* 7000 BC), a pre-pottery Neolithic settlement in the Jordan valley, Diana Kirkbride described 'tens of thousands of grain impressions' in the burnt plaster floor of a building which had been destroyed by fire (Kirkbride 1968, 267). This is an intriguing description. Hoes, sickles, quern stones, stone bowls and bitumen-lined baskets attest to the cultivation, harvesting and processing of grain, perhaps making malt and malt sugars. At Tell Ramad in Syria, *c.* 7000 BC, sickle blades, stone bowls and quern stones were found, as well as grain storage silos, hearths, ovens and 'lime plastered floors with an upturned edge' (de Contenson 1971, 282). The upturned edge would contain the malt as it was raked and turned.

Garfinkel (1987) discusses the use of lime plaster for floors, walls and waterproof baskets. He explains the complex process of making lime plaster, noting that the floor at Ain Ghazal, *c.* 7000 BC, was re-plastered five times (*ibid*. 72). Why were these smooth, level floors so important to the early grain processors? The possibility that some of them were used as malting floors must be considered.

The Craft of the Maltster

Drying the malt

In a consistent hot, dry climate it is possible to dry malt in the sun. Facilities suitable for the drying of malt have been found at settlement sites of the Fertile Crescent from the eighth millennium BC onwards. At Ali Kosh, 7200–6400 BC, domed mud-brick ovens and brick-lined 'roasting pits' were found (Maisels 1990). At Jarmo, an early Neolithic site in the Zagros Mountains, features described as 'baked in place basins' were found. These were described as ovoid depressions, with rims coated with heavily plant-tempered clayey mud and burnished, before being subjected to fire. 'Oven-like structures' were also described (Braidwood et al. 1983). Helbaek (in Braidwood 1983) suggested that these were used for dehusking wild grain, a task he believed most easily achieved on a hot surface. He argued that a well-smoothed floor was necessary for whatever use was being made of these features (Braidwood 1983, 157).

The 'baked in place basins' and 'oven-like structures' may have been used for drying malt. A fire was lit on the surface, then cleared away when it was hot enough to dry the malt. Grain drying for storage could also have been associated with these features. By the third millennium BC oven-like features like these, with fire-hardened inner surfaces, were a common feature of settlements in the Near East and their interpretation for drying grain is generally accepted (Braidwood et al. 1983, 157). Perhaps some of the grain that they were drying was malted.

Archaeological evidence for malted grains

Desiccated grains from Amarna, Egypt, dated to the second millennium BC, were examined using a scanning electron microscope and identified as malt (Palmer 1995; Samuel 1996). It was observed that the husk and aleurone layer were separated from the underlying starchy endosperm, as usually occurs in well-malted barley. Individual starch granules were eroded by enzymatic activity. These are clear signs that the grain had begun to germinate.

During excavations at Balbridie, Fife, Scotland, the site of a large rectangular timber building dated to *c.* 4000 BC, thousands of carbonized grains were found (Fairweather and Ralston 1993). In 2002, I was given six of these grains to examine. One was photographed using a scanning electron microscope (Figure 5.3). The embryo is very neatly missing. Some of the other grains also had missing embryos, clearly visible under a microscope. This neat detachment of the embryo is intriguing. How could this be done using a saddle quern? It could indicate processing by deliberate germination or malting. Further investigation of more samples of carbonized grain is necessary.

Carbonized grain, some whole, some fragmented and some with missing embryos, is found at several rectangular timber buildings dated to the Neolithic in the British Isles. Are some of these discoveries of damaged carbonized grain indicative of malting? At Tankardstown, Co. Limerick, Ireland, *c.* 4000–3300 BC, organic material included hazelnuts, dried wild apples, crab-apple seeds and carbonized grain (Gowan 1988). There were 43 whole grains and 32 fragments. All had missing embryos. Glumes and spikelets

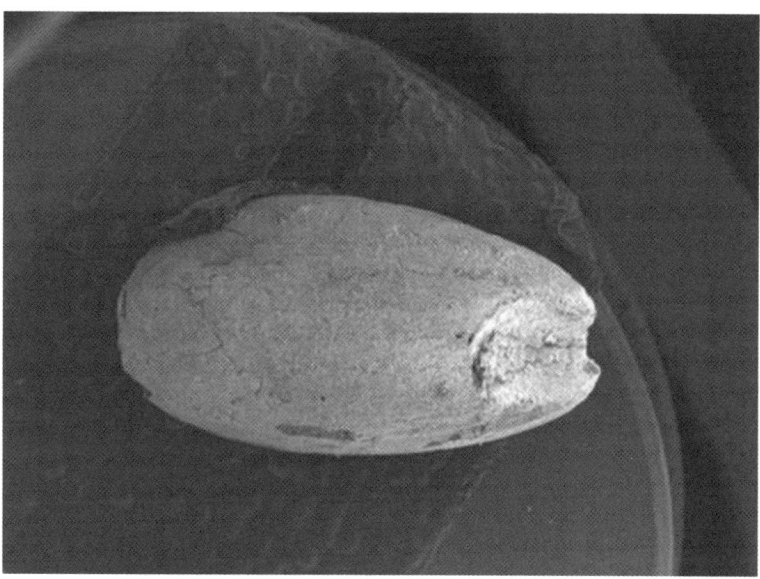

Figure 5.3: Scanning Electric Microscope image of a carbonized grain, with missing embryo visible on the right, from Balbridie, Fife, Scotland. The excavation of this rectangular timber building, dated to c. 4000 BC, uncovered thousands of grains.w (Photo taken as part of funding applications between 2000 and 2004. Courtesy of the Satake Centre for Grain Process Engineering, University of Manchester.)

were found around the building. This archaeobotanical evidence indicates threshing, winnowing and, maybe, malting and brewing. The surviving floor of the rectangular timber building was made of beaten earth and therefore suitable as a malting floor. There was an area of oxidized clay, indicating the site of a hearth or oven, bowl sherds and burnt animal bone. Such archaeological evidence suggests malting, brewing and feasting.

In recent excavations at Ronaldsway, Isle of Man, whole and fragmented carbonized grains were found by flotation (Darvill 1996). These cereal remains were deemed 'unsuitable for flour' (Darvill 1996, 37). Perhaps they represent a failed malt kilning. Flint blades with sickle gloss and grinding stones attest to the cultivation and processing of grain at this Neolithic site. The floor of the rectangular timber building was described as a level area of beaten earth, curving upwards towards the wall and terminating abruptly (Bruce et al. 1947, 145). Was this used as a malting floor? It is perfectly suitable.

Conclusion

In 1953, Braidwood initiated the now famous debate about 'Bread or Beer', discussing with several anthropologists and archaeologists the probable reasons for the origin of grain agriculture in the Fertile Crescent. This debate is important within archaeology and anthropology. It has continued for over half a century and is a complex issue (Smith 1998; Cohen et al. 2009). It seems that the maltster's craft dates back to these early agricultural times.

The processing of grain to make malt was an important incentive for the early agriculturalists (Braidwood 1953; Katz and Voigt 1986; Katz and Maytag 1991; Steinkraus 1995, 407; Dineley 2004). Malting is likely to have been discovered in the late Epipalaeolithic, when people began to harvest and process wild wheat and barley in the Fertile Crescent, over ten thousand years ago. Malted grain is nutritious and much easier to crush than unmalted grain. If the first agriculturalists allowed their grain, either barley or wheat, to grow slightly prior to crushing, they could have made fermentable malt sugars very easily, by gently heating crushed malt with water. They would have made a sweet mash, not a starchy gruel or porridge. Malt sugars have a sweet, delicious taste that is still popular today.

The knowledge and skills necessary to transform inedible grain into sweetness in the form of malt and malt sugars may have been learned at the dawn of grain agriculture and may have been a primary reason for the origin of grain agriculture.

Acknowledgements

Thanks are due to Ivor Murrell, Director General (retired) of the Maltster's Association of Great Britain for his support, encouragement and detailed comments on early drafts of this paper. His knowledge as a professional maltster is invaluable. I also thank Harry Flett, Custodian (retired) of the Corrigall Farm Museum, Orkney, for discussions of historic malting techniques in the early years of my research. Finally, many thanks to Dr Severino Pandiella of UMIST, Manchester. The scanning electron microscope image of the Balbridie grain could not have been done without his assistance and support.

References

Bennett, J. 1996. *Ale, Beer and Brewsters in England: Women's work in a changing world*, Oxford.
Bewley, J. and Black, M. 1994. *Seeds: Physiology of development and germination*, New York.
Braidwood, R. 1953. 'Did Man once live by Bread alone?' *American Anthropologist* 55, 515–526.
Braidwood, L.S., Braidwood, R. J., Howe, B., Reed, C. A., and Watson, P.J. (eds.) 1983. *Prehistoric Archaeology along the Zagros Flanks*, Chicago.
Briggs, D. 1998. *Malt and Malting*, London.
Bruce, M., Megaw, E.M., and Megaw, B.R.S. 1947. 'A Neolithic site at Ronaldsway, Isle of Man', *Proceedings of the Prehistoric Society* 13, 139–160.
Civil, M. 1964. 'A Hymn to the Beer Goddess and a Drinking Song', in Biggs, R.D. and Brinkan, J.A. (eds.), *From the Workshop of the Chicago Assyrian Dictionary: Studies presented to A. Leo Oppenheim: June 7 1964*, Chicago, 67–89.
Cohen, M., Hayden, B., Lambert, P., Gage T., DeWitte, S., Gremillion, K. and Piperno, D. 2009. 'Rethinking the Origins of Agriculture', *Current Anthropology* 50(5), 587–649.
Cobbett, W. 2007 [1821]. *Cottage Economy*, New York.
Darvill, T. 1996. *Billown Neolithic Landscape Project, Isle of Man 1995*, (Bournemouth University School of Conservation Sciences Research Report 1), Bournemouth.

de Contenson, H. 1971. 'Tell Ramad, a village of Syria of the 7th and 6th Millennia BC', *Archaeology* 24, 278–285.
Dineley, M. 2000. 'Neolithic Ale: Barley as a source of sugars for fermentation', in Fairbairn, A.S. (ed.), *Plants in the Neolithic and Beyond*, Oxford, 137–153.
Dineley, M. 2004. *Barley Malt and Ale in the Neolithic*', BAR International Series 1213, Oxford.
Fairweather, A. and Ralston, I. 1993. 'The Neolithic timber hall at Balbridie, Grampian Region, Scotland: A preliminary note on dating and plant macrofossils', *Antiquity* 67, 313–323.
Firth, J. 1922. *Reminiscences of an Orkney Parish*, Stromness.
Garfinkel, Y. 1987. 'Burnt Lime products and social implications in the pre-pottery Neolithic villages of the Near East', *Palaeorient* 13(1), 69–73.
Gowen, M. 1988. *Three Irish Gas Pipelines: New archaeological evidence from Munster*, Dublin.
Hornsey, I. 2003. *A History of Beer and Brewing*, Cambridge.
Hough, J. 1985. *The Biotechnology of Malting and Brewing*, Cambridge Studies in Biotechnology 1, Cambridge.
Katz, S. and Voigt, M. 1986. 'Bread and Beer: The early use of cereals in the human diet', *Expedition* 25(2), 23–34.
Katz, S. and Maytag, F. 1991. 'Brewing an Ancient Beer', *Archaeology* 44(4), 24–33.
Kirkbride, D. 1968. 'Beidha: Early Neolithic Village Life South of the Dead Sea', *Antiquity* 42(168), 263–274.
Kistemaker, R.E. and van Vilsteren, V.T. 1994. *Beer! The Story of Holland's favourite drink*, Amsterdam.
Line, D. 1985. *The Big Book of Brewing*, Michigan.
Maisels, K. 1990. *The Emergence of Civilisation*, London.
Murrell, I. 2006. Malt – Unravelling the mystery. www.ukmalt.com/node/107
Murrell, I. 2006. Personal communication with the author.
Palmer, G. 1995. 'Structure of Ancient Cereal Grains', *Journal of the Institute of Brewing* 101, 103–112.
Samuel, D. 1996. 'Archaeology of Ancient Egyptian Beer', *Journal of the American Society of Brewing Chemists* 54(1), 3–12.
Steinkraus, K. 1995. *Handbook of indigenous fermented foods,* New York.
Stopes, H. 1885. *Malt and Malting, an Historical Scientific and Practical Treatise*, London.
Smith, B. 1998. *The Emergence of Agriculture,* New York.
van Loon, M. 1968. 'The Oriental Institute Excavations at Mureybit, Syria: Preliminary Report on the 1965 Campaign', *Journal of Near Eastern Studies* 27(4), 265–290.

Pottery as Evidence for Lifestyles in Early Iron Age Corinthia (c. 1100–690 BC): Water, Commensality and Ownership

Sam Farnham
University of Nottingham

Dedicated to the memory of Gail Wright

Study area

Table 6.1. Absolute and relative dates of the periods mentioned in the text (Coldstream 2008; Deger-Jalkotzy 2008, 392–393, Fig.1.1 with references).

Relative date	Abbreviation	Chronology (BC)
Bronze Age	BA	3100–1190
Early Iron Age	EIA	1100–690
Late Proto-Geometric	LPG	900–875
Early Geometric	EG	875–825
Middle Geometric I	MG I	825–800
Middle Geometric II	MG II	800–750
Late Geometric	LG	750–720
Early Proto-Corinthian	EPC	720–690

The region of the Corinthia is situated in the north-east Peloponnese where occupation is attested as far back as Early Neolithic times, the middle of the seventh millennium BC (Lavezzi 2003). Despite Bronze Age (see Table 6.1) occupation being sparse in relation to other regions of Greece, the suggestion that by the fifteenth century BC most of the Corinthia was ruled by Mycenae is supported by a road network that links Corinth to Mycenae and Kleonai in the south-west and the absence of monumental tomb architecture (Cherry and Davis 2001, 156, Fig.10.1). Mycenaean states existed during the fourteenth and thirteenth centuries BC in Greece and even if Mycenae had annexed the Corinthia, the political and economic status of the region is unclear from the extant administrative documents in Linear B script. For the twelfth century BC, the post-palatial period, there are sizeable settlement deposits from Korakou (Blegen 1921), the site of the later sanctuary of Demeter and Kore (Rutter 1979) and some graves near Corinth itself, but evidence for EIA settlement is sparse until LPG (Salmon 1984, Fig.7). Inhumation burials are clustered around Corinth and much pottery is dedicated in sanctuary contexts at Isthmia, c. 5 km to the east (Morgan 1999). Later literary evidence suggests that the area was ruled by an oligarchy, the Bacchiads, who were usurped by the tyrant Cypselus in 657 BC. The exact date of the oligarchy's inception is not clear from the extant textual sources, the historian Diodorus Siculus writing in the first century BC states:

> The Bacchiads, descendants of Heracles, were more than 200 in number and held authority; all of them ruled the city in common, and for ninety years until the tyranny of Cypselus, who overthrew them, they chose each year one of their number to be prytanis and exercise the functions of the king. (Quoted from Salmon 1984, 56)

Strabo, an ancient geographer writing in the first century BC, even suggests the Bacchiads reigned for 200 years prior to Cypselus. Yet as Salmon points out (1984, 56) in his study of Corinth from the earliest occupation until 338 BC, the accurate preservation of any such chronology during and after subsequent regimes of such contrasting political difference is unlikely.

Oligarchic commensality could be expected to fit into Dietler's (2001, 85–88) category of the 'diacritical feast', with an elite practice of consumption, preparation and service that could be expected to be evident in the pottery, differentiating the aristocrats from the rest of the populace. Can the archaeological evidence for commensality throw any light upon the opaque picture of political organization in EIA Corinthia?

Methodology

Pottery is quantified from two ritual contexts, burial and sanctuary, by dividing the number for each functional category at each specific date by the total number for each specific date to obtain a percentage. Function is assigned to pottery on the basis of shape, size and surface modification, though a lack of burning on the surface of a vessel does not necessarily mean it was not used for cooking (Moore 2010, esp. 44, 47). The force of my argument can withstand a margin of error between shapes in the smaller functional categories, in particular cooking, eating and storage, since they form such small statistical proportions when compared with drinking and pouring vessels from all contexts. This analysis is subject to periods where sufficient sample size is available so although it is not possible to always compare all find-contexts this is unavoidable.

Analysis

Burial

In terms of the pots deposited in burials, Figure 6.1 shows there is a staggered rise in drinking and a more drastic decrease in pouring *c.* 875–690 BC. This is accompanied by a widespread decrease in pottery deposited in graves from the middle of the eighth century onwards, part of a change in burial rite to investing wealth in the monolithic sarcophagi rather than grave goods (Dickey 1992, 103; Pfaff 2007, 530). The vital point

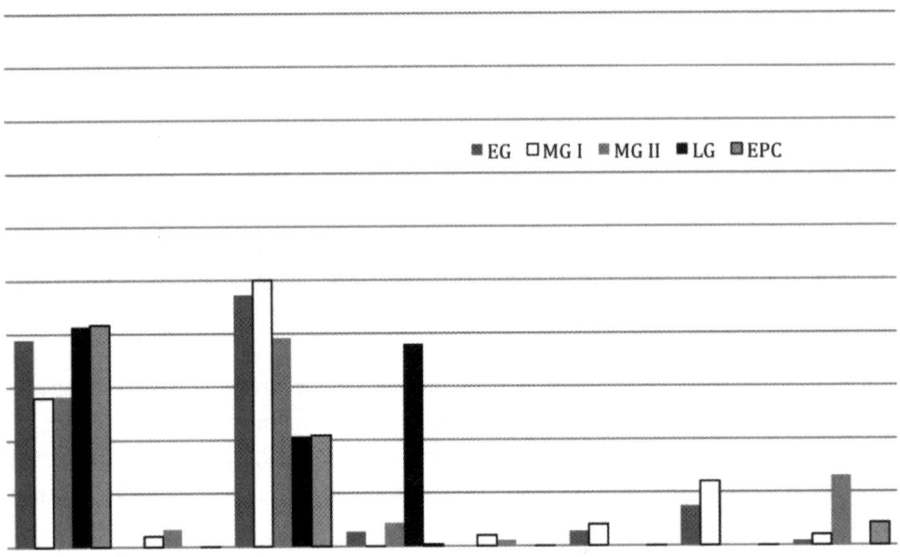

Pottery as Evidence for Lifestyles in Early Iron Age Corinthia

Figure 6.1. Pottery deposited in burial contexts classified by function as percentages 875–690 BC (data taken from Lawrence 1964; Pfaff 1999, 2007; Stillwell and Benson 1984; Weinberg 1943, 1948, 1974; Williams 1970; Williams et al. 1974; Charitonides 1955, 1957; Hill 1927; Nichols 1905; Young 1964; Morgan 1937).

is the eighth century – the sharp increase in drinking preparation vessels (kraters) is preceded by an increase in the deposition of hydriai, which I argue to be water pots – and this change is very important for understanding the 'burial package' that developed at Corinth in the eighth century.

Water pots
It has been suggested that the coarse Corinthian hydriai contained liquids on the grounds that the vessels found in the North Cemetery were covered at the mouth by skyphoi, two-handled bowls (Dickey 1992, 72). These bowls may have been intended as dispensers for the very liquids that they contained. Alternatively, Salmon (1984, 88) considers the Corinthian MG II and LG coarse hydriai at the site of Delphi situated in the valley of Phocis to have been empty wine-jugs. The contextual evidence from the settlement sphere supports the interpretation that they contained water, at least for the hydriai found in Corinth. A well has been discovered below the eastern isle of the cryptoporticus of the South Basilica at Corinth with a use deposit 1m in depth from the bottom dating from LG–EPC (Weinberg 1949, 153–4). Coarse hydriai, morphologically similar to those from the North Cemetery, are estimated to run into 'dozens' of complete vessels: clearly the most frequent shape in this deposit (Weinberg 1949, 153). Further

emphasis on the functional significance of the water pots is their subfusc appearance and coarse fabric: a stark contrast to the fine-ware counterparts from EIA Knossos on Crete (Coldstream 1996, 340–1).

The north cemetery
The North Cemetery at Corinth was used for burial for the first time in at least eight centuries during the first half of the eighth century BC (Young 1964, 13). This regeneration of a place previously reserved for burial was marked by the use of an assemblage where water pots were prominent grave goods for adults. A single water pot was deposited outside each of the three earliest adult graves in the cemetery: Graves 14A, 15A and 16. Accompanied by two child burials, Graves 14B and 15B, these graves were enclosed by a wall (*peribolos*) 8.6 m long and 3.9 m wide on the interior and *c.* 10–15 cm thought to have been visible above the surface during the use of the cemetery (Young 1964, 21). Figure 6.2 can be seen then as a recognition of the symbolic importance of water when the new burial ground was established in MG II, along with pouring and drinking vessels. Indeed, a similar pattern appears to be evident in the Lechaion Road Valley, the site of the Classical Agora, located in central Corinth. Grave D, and Graves A and B had a coarse hydriai closed by bronze vessels stood outside, and a further example of this was found at the west end of the valley, probably contemporary on the grounds of rite (Weinberg 1943, 25–28; Coldstream 2008, 95–98, n. 1; Dickey 1992, A–3 no. LV–6). This was followed in LG by a dramatic increase in the types of vessel used to mix water with wine. Though the many large kraters in the latter period have been interpreted as containing child burials, in only one instance were bones found within a vessel: in the case of Grave 44, no. 44–1 (Young 1964, 34), so the argument from silence is weak. It is more probable the kraters held the remains of graveside meals honouring the dead.

Funerals and the community
The key to understanding the deposition of grave goods is their context relative to the settlement and sanctuaries. The actual act of burial would have probably been conducted by a restricted social group in contrast to the more public deposition in open-air sanctuaries. For the former, the crucial point in the different stages of corpse disposal is between the corpse lying in state on a bier/bed (*prothesis*) and the act of transporting the body to its resting place (*ekphora*) (see Garland 1985, 23–31, Fig. 6, 31–34, Fig. 8). In contrast to other contemporary and earlier burials made within the area of settlement (Pfaff 2007, 445, 529), the reservation of a separate place for burial outside a settlement may have made funerary rites more conspicuous events to onlookers, perhaps due to an increased emphasis on processions at funerals.

Sanctuaries
In the sanctuary contexts illustrated in Figure 6.2, drinking vessels dominate the pottery from the inception of the sanctuary *c.* 900 BC, which is maintained for a

Pottery as Evidence for Lifestyles in Early Iron Age Corinthia

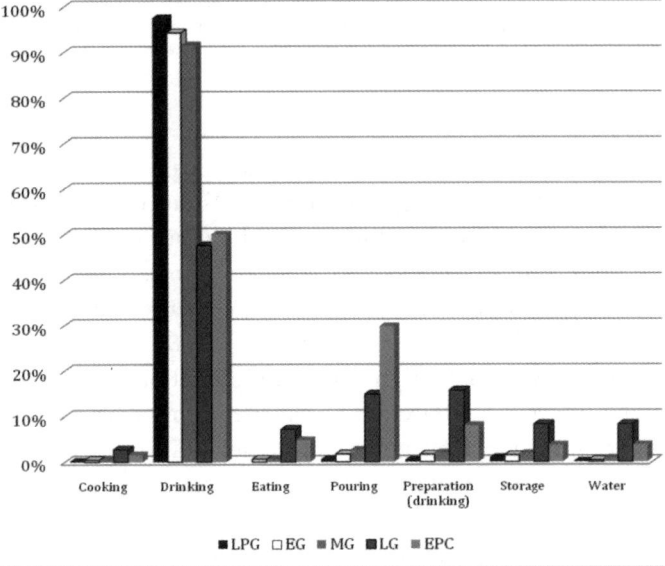

Figure 6.2. Pottery deposited in sanctuary contexts classified by function as percentages 900–690 BC (data taken from Morgan 1999; Pfaff 1998; Broneer 1958: 29; Payne 1940; Robinson 1976).

period of 125 years. In contrast to the settlement and burial, there is no elaboration in the range of pottery functions until LG, when many components of which: drinking, pouring, preparation (drinking), water and probably storage too, imply an emphasis on broadening the ceramic repertoire in relation to drinking and perhaps also libation rites.

Interpretation: Property rights

The natural environment

The symbolic recognition of water as part of burial happened concomitantly with an increase in the use of wells. The significance of this is enhanced by the multitude of natural water sources in the Corinthia, which are situated within 1 km of the area of settlement (Landon 2003, Fig.3)(Figure 6.3). Knowledge of this in antiquity is supported by a funerary inscription from the island of Salamis in the Saronic Gulf west of Athens commemorating Corinthians who died during the Persian Wars early in the fifth century BC, which noted Corinth as 'well-watered', and also from a literary source: the second century AD traveller Pausanias praised the Romans for founding a colony here due to the abundance of natural water supplies (Landon 2003, 43, n.3; Salmon 1984, 255). Given the evidence from the pottery, the need to undertake the labour-intensive task of accessing further supplies of potable water in such close proximity to natural supplies, water seems to have increased in value as a resource during MG II. The

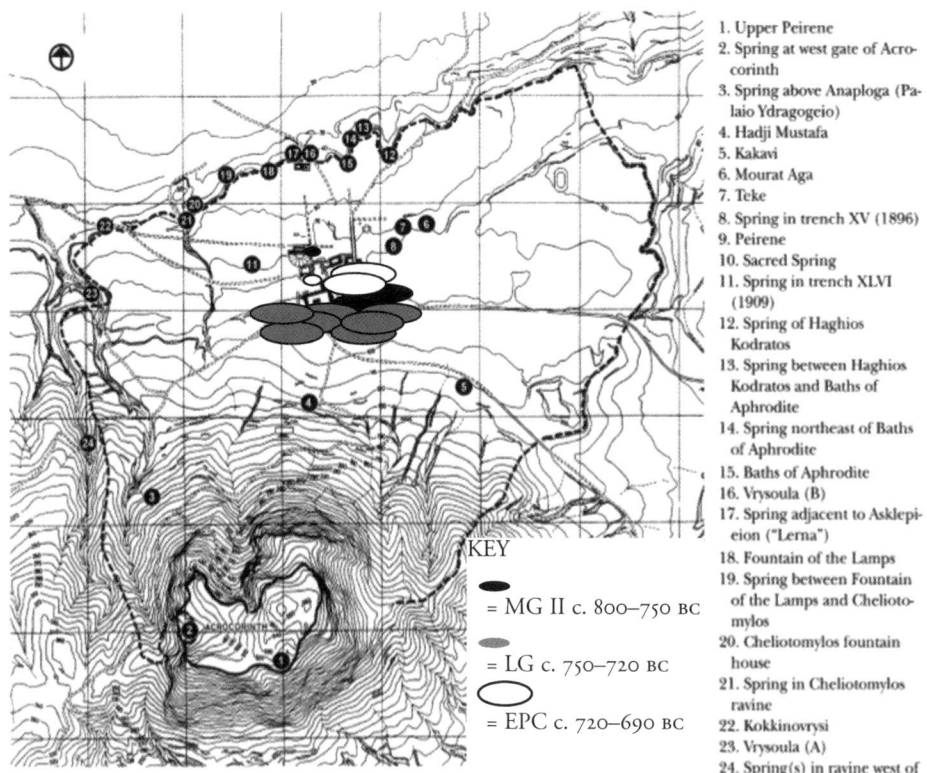

Figure 6.3: Topographical map of the natural water sources in Corinth and the 8th and 7th century wells with some post-EIA structures. Wells with pottery dating to two subsequent periods have been dated to the earliest period (after Landon 2003, Fig. 3.1 using Pfaff 1988, Fig.2).

distribution of wells in LG and EPC implies that this process intensified during LG, an argument again supported by the pottery used for water from both burials and the sanctuaries. This process seems to have reduced in intensity during EPC.

Ownership
One possible explanation for this rise in private supplies of water is an accentuated perception of property ownership. The overseas colonies founded by Corinth during the 730s have also been understood in terms of strains on the land (Salmon 1984, 62–67). This chronology for colonization has been confirmed by the local, non-Greek archaeology at Syracuse in Sicily, which affirms the date offered by the military historian Thucydides and perhaps gives support to a similar situation at the less-explored site of Corcyra on the modern island of Corfu (Salmon 1984, 62, n.34). The wells and the

emphasis on water indicated by the use of water pots in the North Cemetery suggest that political tensions over private property rights was a long-term factor that contributed towards the desire for colonization. The increase in the number of new wells in LG, contemporary with the vast increase in the deposition of kraters and drinking vessels in burials and a broadening of the pottery assemblage in the sanctuary, argues for an intensification of the demand on water in fulfilling both private and public exigencies at this point. This process seems to have decreased by EPC: perhaps by this point property rights were less contested due to the impact of colonization?

Ethnography
The above suggestion finds further support in the ethnographic record. In his study of the physiological implications of water, Vargas (2001, 15) concluded that despite natural supplies, population increase resulted in water becoming scarce as a resource. It is tempting to follow this line of argument here, but it would fail to account for both the symbolic recognition of water pots in the North Cemetery and the diversification in the ceramic repertoire observed in the sanctuary. Pollock, in her study of the Marshall Islands in the Pacific, found that access to water was determined by ownership of the territory by certain social groups that had a well, coconut tree or cistern within its territory (Pollock 2001, 46–7). Of these, only wells are known for Corinth, which is heightened in value since 40 cm annual rainfall makes the site one of the driest in the Peloponnese (Landon 2003, 43). When it does rain it occurs in large bursts for short periods of time (Salmon 1984, 8). Water obtained by other means, such as the collection of rainwater in pots fulfilling a secondary function, would probably constitute only a small amount of the water used on a daily basis. The majority of EIA Corinthians' water probably came from wells and natural water sources as they fell within land boundaries of property, perhaps organized by household.

Conclusions

It probably stretches the evidence to suggest that the inception of an aristocracy can be directly observed archaeologically from a ceramic perspective. The foundation of the North Cemetery fails to confirm either literary testimony. Yet it is possible to identify aspects of ownership, which would probably have conferred political power through wealth distributed between separate social groups. The need to undertake the labour-intensive task of accessing further supplies of potable water in such close proximity to natural supplies, suggests that land ownership and access-rights intensified during the first half of the eighth century BC. This intensification was accentuated during LG, though became alleviated hereafter. Ownership of a water supply was a requirement for the practice of culturally important observances and it was also of course a physiological necessity. The nascent importance of the role of water was symbolically recognized by the burying groups that founded and subsequently used the North Cemetery and those burying elsewhere in Corinth. Later intensification during LG seems to have been focussed in the context of drinking and libations and was also prominent in the public sphere. Water may well have been of further value in cooking and cleansing yet the data suggest these factors were of a lesser relative importance for pottery use. The question raised regarding the relationship between burial and sanctuary will be pursued in a future paper (Farnham, forthcoming).

Acknowledgements

Prof. Alan Outram very kindly brought my attention to and sent me a copy of Jeremy Moore's MA Dissertation, for which I express further gratitude to the author, in addition to that for his permission to cite it in my PhD and arising publications. I am particularly grateful to Bill Cavanagh for providing many comments on an earlier draft of this paper and for his diligent supervision of my PhD thesis from which this study arose. Nevertheless, any errors that remain are my fault alone.

References

Blegen, C.W. 1928. *Zygouries a prehistoric settlement in the valley of Cleonae*, Cambridge, Mass.
Blegen, C.W. 1921. *Korakou: A Prehistoric Settlement near Corinth*, Boston.
Broneer, O. 1958. 'Excavations at Isthmia: Third Campaign, 1955–1956', *Hesperia* 26, 1–37.
Charitonides, S. 1955. 'A Geometric Grave at Clenia in Corinthia', *American Journal of Archaeology* 59, 125–28.
Charitonides, S. 1957. 'More Geometric from the Corinthia', *American Journal of Archaeology* 61, 169–171.
Cherry, J.F. and Davis, J.L. 2001. 'Under the Sceptre of Agamemnon: The View from the Hinterlands of Mycenae', in Branigan, K. (ed.), *Urbanism in the Aegean Bronze Age*. (Sheffield Studies in Aegean Archaeology 4), London/New York, 141–59.
Coldstream, J.N. 2008. *Greek Geometric pottery. A survey of ten local styles and their chronology*. Second Edition, Bristol.
Coldstream, J.N. 1996. 'The protogeometric and geometric pottery', in Coldstream, J.N. and Catling, H.W. (eds.), *Knossos North Cemetery. Vol. II: Discussion*, London, 311–420.
Deger-Jalkotzy, S. 2008. 'Decline, Destruction, Aftermath', in Shelmerdine, C. (ed.), *The Cambridge Companion to the Aegean Bronze Age*, New York, 387–415.
Dickey, K. 1992. *Corinthian burial customs ca. 1100–500 BC*, PhD Diss. Bryn Mawr College.
Dietler, M. 2001. 'Theorizing the Feast: Rituals of Consumption, Commensal Politics, and Power in African Contexts', in Dietler, M. and Hayden, B. (eds.), *Feasts: Archaeological and Ethnographic Perspectives on Food, Politics and Power*, Washington, 65–114.
Farnham, S. Forthcoming. 'Interplay between burial and sanctuary? Sacrifice and the use of water in the Argolid and Corinthia during the Early Iron Age', in *Sacred landscapes in the Peloponnese from Prehistory to post-Byzantine times. Proceedings of the Third CSPS International Conference, 30/3–1/4/2012*, Sparta/Nottingham.
Garland, R. 1985. *The Greek Way of Death*, London.
Hill, B.H. 1927. 'Excavations at Corinth, 1926', *American Journal of Archaeology* 31, 70–79.
Lawrence, P. 1964. 'Five Grave Groups from the Corinthia', *Hesperia* 33, 89–107.
Landon, M.E. 2003. 'Beyond Peirene: Towards a Broader View of Corinthian Water Supply', in Williams, C.K. II and Bookidis, N. (eds.), *Corinth Vol. 20, The Centenary: 1896–1996*, Princeton, 43–62.
Lavezzi, J.C. 2003. 'Corinth before the Mycenaeans', in Williams, C.K. II and Bookidis, N. (eds.), *Corinth Vol. 20, The Centenary: 1896–1996*, Princeton, 63–74.

Moore, J. 2010. *Pot-Boiling versus Direct Firing: An experimental exploration of prehistoric heating practices.* Masters Diss. University of Exeter.

Morgan, C. 1999. *Isthmia VIII: The Late Bronze Age Settlement and Early Iron Age Sanctuary,* Princeton.

Morgan, C.H. II. 1937. 'Excavations at Corinth, 1936–1937', *American Journal of Archaeology* 41, 539–552.

Nichols, M. 1905. 'Geometric Vases from Corinth', *American Journal of Archaeology* 9, 411–421.

Pfaff, C. 2007. 'Geometric Graves in the Panayia Field at Corinth', *Hesperia* 76, 443–537.

Pfaff, C. 1998. 'The Early Iron Age Pottery from the Sanctuary of Demeter and Kore at Corinth', *Hesperia* 67, 55–134.

Pfaff, C.A. 1988. 'A Geometric Well at Corinth: Well 1981–6', *Hesperia* 57, 21–80.

Pollock, N.J. 2001. '4. Nor Any Drop to Drink: Everyday Drinking Habits in Pacific and New Zealand Societies', in de Garine, I. and de Garine, V. (eds.), *Drinking Anthropological Approaches,* New York/Oxford, 35–50.

Robinson, H.S. 1976. 'Excavations at Corinth: Temple Hill, 1968–1972', *Hesperia* 45, 203–39.

Rutter, J. 1979. 'The Last Mycenaeans at Corinth', *Hesperia* 48, 348–392.

Salmon, J.B. 1984. *Wealthy Corinth. A history of the city to 338 BC,* Oxford.

Stillwell, A.N. and Benson, G.L. 1984, *Corinth XV, iii: The Potters' Quarter,* Princeton.

Vargas, J.L. 2001. '2. Thirst and Drinking as a Biocultural Process', in de Garine, I. and de Garine, V. (eds.), *Drinking Anthropological Approaches,* New York/Oxford, 11–21.

Weinberg, S.S. 1974. 'ΚΤΛ from Corinth', *Hesperia* 43, 522–534.

Weinberg, S.S. 1949. 'Investigations at Corinth, 1947–1948', *Hesperia* 18, 148–157.

Weinberg, S.S. 1948. 'A cross-section of Corinthian Antiquities', *Hesperia* 17, 197–241.

Weinberg, S.S. 1943. *Corinth VII, i: The Geometric and Orientalizing Pottery,* Cambridge, Mass.

Williams, C.K. II. 1970. 'Corinth, 1969: Forum Area', *Hesperia* 39, 1–39.

Williams, C.K. II and Fisher, J.E. 1971. 'Corinth, 1972: The Forum Area', *Hesperia* 42, 1–44.

Williams, C.K. II, Macintosh, J. and Fisher, J.E. 1974. 'Excavations at Corinth, 1973', *Hesperia* 43, 1–73.

Young, R.S. 1964. 'Part II', in Blegen, C.W. (ed.), *Corinth XIII: The North Cemetery,* Princeton, 13–49.

The Preliminary Results from a Herculaneum Sewer: What's Inside? Why? And what Can it Tell us about Roman Diet?

Erica Rowan
University of Oxford

The town of Herculaneum, along with Pompeii and numerous villas, was buried during the eruption of Mount Vesuvius in AD 79. Herculaneum's unique state of preservation makes it one of the best sites where ancient Roman diet can be studied using environmental archaeology. This paper examines the biological contents of the Cardo V sewer lying beneath *Insula Orientalis* II (Figure 7.1). The food remains are in an excellent state of preservation for three primary reasons. Firstly, the eruption of Vesuvius buried Herculaneum under many metres of pyroclastic flows, protecting the sewer from the elements and organic interference. Secondly, the contents of the sewer itself have aided enormously in the preservation process and thirdly, the geology around and beneath the town, which led to the construction of the sewer.

Herculaneum rests on a seaward sloping terrace that had a stream bed on either side (Jansen 1991, 146). Unlike the porous volcanic subsoil of Pompeii, Herculaneum sits on hard, compact tuff. This helps to explain why the smaller, less populated town of Herculaneum had four large underground sewers while Pompeii had primarily soakaway latrines. The porous soil in Pompeii meant that the waste water emptied into a cess pit would quickly leach away into the ground, allowing for the long-term use of these pits (Jansen 2000, 38–44). In Herculaneum the tuff did not absorb water and instead, during the pre-Augustan period, a sewer was built under Cardo III (Jansen 1991, 160).

Later, during the reign of Augustus, the town was connected to an aqueduct (Camardo 2006, 184).[1] Once the town had a piped water supply, a *palaestra* with a large swimming pool was constructed in the eastern section of the town, during the first quarter of the first century AD (Monteix 2010, 257–260; Jansen 1991, 160). The construction of the *palaestra* was subsidized by building *Insula Orientalis* II, a long stretch of connected buildings with shops on the ground floor and apartments above which would yield rent (Wallace-Hadrill 1994, 117). The *insula* is located adjacent to the *palaestra* and Cardo V. The perfect alignment of the latrines in the shops and apartments of *Insula Orientalis* II demonstrates that the Cardo V sewer was built at the same time as the shops and *palaestra*.

The Cardo V sewer has two main branches; a north-south branch running beneath

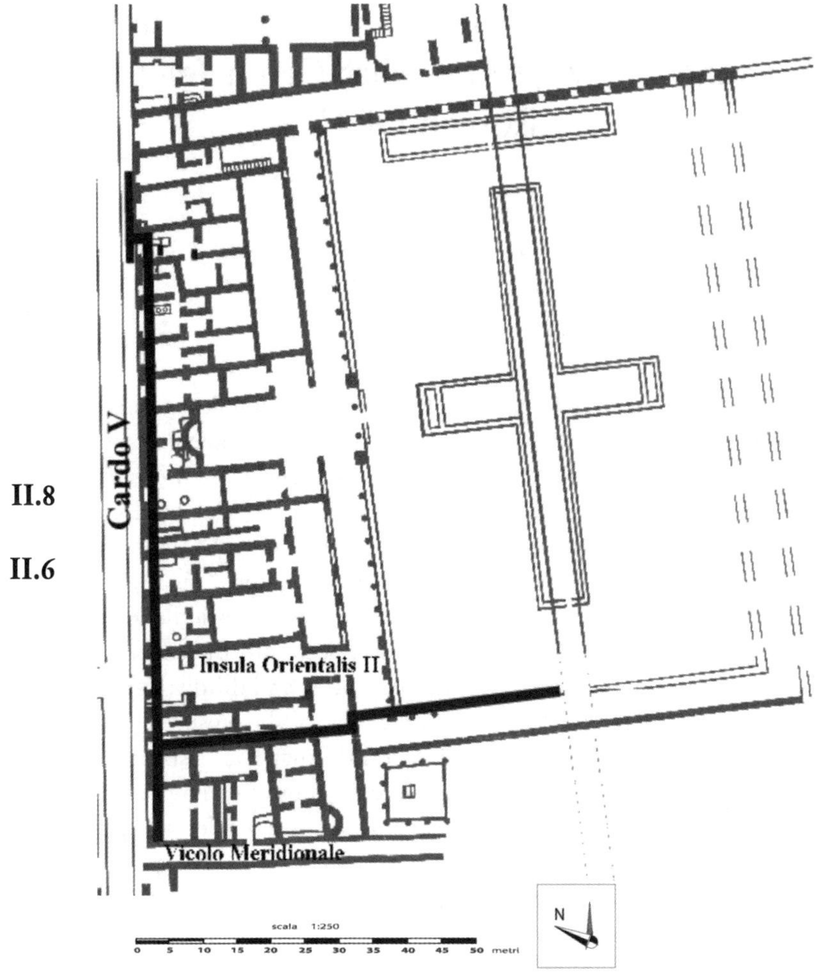

Figure 7.1: Plan. Insula Orientalis II and the Cardo V sewer (Sosandra/HCP). The north-south branch runs parallel to the Cardo V.

the façade of the insula and an east-west branch running perpendicular to it designed to clear water away from the *palaestra* and presumably drain its *piscina* (Figure 7.1). The branch that runs under the shops, the one excavated in this study, is 0.8m wide and 0.8m high with the height slowly increasing to 3.6m. The walls were built in *opus incertum* or *reticulatum* and were lined with cement (Camadro 2006, 187–188).

The preservation of the sewer contents is primarily due to the L-shaped design of the sewer complex. Except for three small roof drains, the sewer did not collect rainwater and was fed exclusively by latrine shafts coming from the shops and apartments (Andrews 2012). Additionally, since the two sewer branches meet at the southern end of

The Preliminary Results from a Herculaneum Sewer

Insula Orientalis II the waste water coming from the *palaestra* would not wash away the contents of the Cardo V branch. Waste water flushed into the Cardo V branch would drain away but the solid contents would remain, turning the sewer into a large cess pit that needed to be cleaned out periodically (Robinson 2007a, 2). When Maiuri explored the sewer in 1949, the deposit was 1.35 m deep, demonstrating that there had been no recent cleaning of the sewer before the time of the eruption (Camardo 2007b, 181).

Methods

Recognizing the unique nature of the Cardo V deposit, the Herculaneum Conservation Project, in association with Professor Mark Robinson, undertook a detailed and systematic excavation of the sewer contents in 2007 (Camardo 2007b, 210). This was done primarily so that the sewer could be used to hold modern pipes to drain water out of the site as it is currently below sea level and is often subject to water damage (Robinson 2007a, 1).

The sewer was divided up into one-metre quadrants running from *Insula Orientalis* II.6 to II.14.[2] The quadrants were subsequently excavated based on the stratigraphy of the whole sewer, with similar layers receiving identical identification numbers. Ten litre samples were taken from every other stratigraphic layer for processing. Flotation (0.5mm mesh) and sieving (2mm and 1mm meshes) were used to separate the lighter materials, such as seeds, from the heavier deposits (Robinson 2007b, 1). The material was brought back to Oxford and seven samples (70L) were sorted by the author using a binocular microscope. The mineralized and carbonized material was identified using Dr Mark Robinson's private seed collection. The identification of the sea shells and sea urchins took place using photographs both from books and the internet as no physical specimens were available for comparison. Identifications were confirmed by Jennifer Robinson.

Study samples

The sample sequences examined in this paper come from Quadrants 3–4 and 13–14. Quadrant 3–4 is situated beneath shop number six of *Insula Orientalis* II (II.6 in Figure 7.1). At the front of the shop there is an L-shaped counter containing four embedded *dolia*. The presence of the counter, combined with the numerous amphorae found stacked at the back, suggests that this shop sold food and drinks (Maiuri 1948, 60). In the south-west corner of the large front room there was a staircase that led to two upper floor rooms. These two rooms extended across the entire length and width of the shop below and had a spacious headroom of 3.4m, suggesting that these rooms acted as the living space for those who owned or worked in the shop below (Andrews 2006, vol 2. 342). A latrine was situated in the south-west corner of the large ground floor room.

To the north, Quadrant 13–14 is situated directly beneath the bakery of Sextus Patulcius Felix (Pesandro 2006, 384) (II.8 in Figure 7.1). The two millstones and an adjacent oven confirm it to be a bakery. A latrine was located in a small side room to the south of the milling room, probably for the benefit of the workers.

Finally, ceramic analysis of the pottery sherds found in the sewer has shown that there was some movement amongst the finds and therefore we cannot directly correlate the finds below a drain to the shop or flat above (Camardo 2006–2007).

Nature of the sewer contents

Although the sample was from a sewer and the material entered the sewer through latrine shafts, not all the biological remains would have passed through the human digestive tract nor were all the items foodstuffs. It was common in Roman houses for latrines to be next to kitchens since they shared a common drain (DeKind 1998, 99). As a result, food preparation waste, such as sea and egg shells were also discarded into the sewer. Aside from the food remains the sewer was inhabited by a variety of insects and other arthropods including latrine flies, sewage flies and woodlice.

It is likely that the vast majority of the plant remains which had become mineralized were consumed. The carbonized plant remains represent either hearth ashes thrown into the latrine or food preparation waste that accidentally fell into the flames.

Nature of preservation

The conditions in the sewer, and its contents, were very conducive to the preservation of biological material. Remains were preserved as carbonized, mineralized, waterlogged and biogenic mineral material, including eggshell, seashell and bone.

In order for an object, for example a seed, to be carbonized it must be heated to 400°C and at some point during the burning process be deprived of oxygen (Mols 1999, 20–21). Carbonization often occurs if the object is covered by hot ash. However, not all the seeds found in the deposit were carbonized. In their study of the AD 79 eruption, Sigurdsson and Carey found both carbonized and uncarbonized wood in the same stratigraphic layer. This signifies that the first pyroclastic surge to hit Herculaneum was not hot enough to cause the full carbonization of exposed organic material. While the surge deposited 1.5 m of ash on the town, the ash which entered the sewer would not have been hot enough to carbonize the organic material in the underlying deposits. Instead, the ash acted like a blanket and protected the contents of the sewer from future carbonization. Wood, however, was fully carbonized in the layer of the second, hotter surge that hit the town (Sigurdsson 2002, 54–55). Therefore, it can be argued that all the carbonized material found in the sewer was carbonized before the eruption.

The mineralization of certain items in the sewer, mostly seeds, was due to the environment of the sewer before the eruption. Seeds become preserved when molecules of calcium phosphate slowly replace the cells of a seed as it decays. This process can also create an internal cast of a seed when the seed embryo decays before the seed coat, leaving a cavity in which calcium phosphate is deposited (Robinson 2006, 212). The human faecal matter in the sewer provided a source of phosphate ions while the calcium carbonate found in items such as egg or seashell supplied the calcium. In addition, common latrine remains such as mammal and fish bones and fish scales can provide both the required phosphate and calcium (Green 1979, 281). In the Cardo V sewer, in addition to the numerous shells and bones present, mortar used in construction and lime used for wall plaster would have acted as additional sources of calcium (Robinson 2006, 214). The circulation of ground water, or in this case, waste water, also helped the mineralization process. The calcareous conditions described above would also have facilitated the preservation of the biogenic material including the fish bones and seashells.

However, not all seeds become mineralized to the same degree and some will simply degrade entirely, even under ideal conditions. Mineralization occurs primarily in seeds that have a permeable coat which allows ions to accumulate in the embryo of the seed (McCobb 2001, 939). The preservation of the embryo unfortunately makes seed identification difficult as the embryo does not always resemble the outer coating of the seed. In addition, broken seeds, such as those ground by milling, do not readily become mineralized (Robinson 2006, 215).

In stratigraphic levels 38 and 40 of Quadrant 13–14 there has been the waterlogged survival of some seeds. Waterlogging occurs when there has been an absence of oxygen (Dincauze 2002, 440). After the eruption, the sewer was sealed off, preventing evaporation and enabling small pockets of material to remain wet until they were excavated in 2007.

Results and discussion

The plant and shell remains from two quadrants have been analysed, yielding 64 different types of plants and 40 shell varieties (Tables 7.1–7.4). The fish and animal bones have only been partially analysed, so they have not been included in this paper. The diversity of food items in these samples has yielded a wealth of information about the diet and lifestyle of those living in *Insula Orientalis* II. Some broad patterns have emerged from the combined samples, such as locality and diversity, and they will be discussed below.

It appears that nearly all of the food consumed by inhabitants of *Insula Orientalis* II was grown, raised or caught locally. Using accounts from the ancient authors, in combination with environmental evidence, it can be confirmed that only one food item, the date seed, could not be found in the Vesuvian area at the time of the eruption (Pliny *NH* 13.26, 42–50; Dalby 2000, 169). The crops and legumes such as wheat and lentil could also have been imported from abroad or grown locally in the Sarno plains. The Murecine tablets, found near Pompeii, record that Alexandrian grain and legumes were being stored in the nearby port town of Puteoli (Rickman 1980, 262–263; Casson 1980). However, aside from the crops, the primary use of local foods attests to the fertility of the region, demonstrates resourcefulness on the part of the inhabitants, and sheds light on their socioeconomic status.

Insula Orientalis II is the only large-scale shop and apartment complex found in the excavated portions of Herculaneum (Wallace-Hadrill 1994, 197–205). Since there is only one large home in *Insula Orientalis* II, apartment II.7, it can be assumed, from

Table 7.1. Mineralized material.

Scientific Name	Common Name	Quantity
cf. *Anethum graveolens* (L.)	Dill	+
Anthemis arvensis (L.)	Corn chamomile	+
Apium graveolens (Mill.)	Celery	+
Boraginaceae	Borage	+
Brassica sp.	Cabbage or Mustard	+
Carex sp.	Sedge	++
Caryophyllaceae	Carnation family	++
cf. *Celtis australis* (L.)	European hackberry	+
Ceratonia siliqua (L.)	Carob	+
Chenopodium sp.	Goose foot	++
Coriandrum sativum (L.)	Coriander	+
Corylus avellana (L.)	Hazelnut	+
Cucumis melo (L.) or *C. sativus* (L.)	Muskmelon or Cucumber	+
Cupressus sempervirens - twig	Cypress	+
Ficus carica (L.)	Fig	+++
cf. *Foeniculum vulgare* (Mill.)	Fennel	++
Gramineae	Wild grass	+
Juncus sp.	Rush	+
Lamiaceae	Mint family	+
Lens culinaris (Medik.)	Lentil	++
cf. *Linum* sp.	Flax	+
Malus or *Pyrus* sp.	Apple or Pear	++
Malva sp.	Mallow	+
Medicago sp.	Medick	+
cf. *Mentha* sp.	Mint	+
Olea europaea (L.)	Olive	+
Ornithopus sp.	Bird's foot	+
Panicum miliaceum (L.)	Broom corn millet	++
Panicum miliaceum (L.) or *Setaria italic* (L.)	Broom corn millet or Italian/foxtail millet	++
Papaver somniferum (L.)	Opium poppy	++
Papaver sp.	Poppy	+
Poaceae	True grasses	+
Polygonum aviculare agg.	Common knotgrass	++

The Preliminary Results from a Herculaneum Sewer

cf. *Polygonum* sp.	Knotgrass	+
cf. *Prunus* sp.	Plum or Cherry	+
Pteridium aquilinum (L.)	Bracken	+
Ranunculus parviflorus (L.)	Small-flowered buttercup	+
Ranunculus sp.	Buttercup	+
Reseda sp.	Mignonette	+
Rubus fruticosus agg.	Blackberry	+
Rumex acetosella agg.	Red/Field sorrel	+
Rumex sp.	Dock	+
Setaria italic (L.)	Italian/foxtail millet	+
Sherardia arvensis (L.)	Field madder	+
Silene gallica (L.)	Small-flowered catchfly	+
Silene sp.	Catchfly	+
Stellaria media (L.)	Common chickweed	+
Stellaria sp.	Chickweed	+
Triticum dicoccum (Schübl.)	Emmer wheat	+
Urtica dioica (L.)	Stinging nettle	+
Urtica sp.	Nettle	++
Umbelliferae	Umbellifers	++
Vicia faba (L.)	Field bean	+
cf. *Vicia* sp.	Vetch	+
Vitis vinifera (L.)	Grape	++

\+ = *MNI 1–10*   ++ = *MNI 11–999*   +++ = *MNI 1000+*
**Results from Quadrants 3–4 and 13–14 have been combined.

Table 7.2. Carbonized material.

Scientific Name	Common Name	Quantity
cf. *Chenopodium* sp.	Goose foot	+
Ficus carica (L.)	Fig	+
Hordeum sp.	Barley	+
Juglans regia (L.)	Common walnut	+
Lens culinaris (Medik.)	Lentil	+
Malus or *Pyrus* sp.	Apple or Pear	+
Olea europaea (L.)	Olive	+++
Phoenix dactylifera (L.)	Date	+
Pinus pinea (L.) - bracts	Stone pine	+

Poaceae	True grasses	+
Pyrus sp.	Pear	+
Setaria italica (L.)	Italian/foxtail millet	+
Stellaria sp.	Chickweed	+
Triticum dicoccum (Schübl.)	Emmer wheat	+
Triticum monococcum (L.) or *Triticum dicoccum* (Schübl.)	Einkorn or emmer wheat	+
Vicia or *Lathyrus* sp.	Vetch or Sweet peas	+
Vitis vinifera (L.)	Grape	++

Table 7.3. Waterlogged material.

Scientific Name	Common Name	Quantity
cf. *Anethum graveolens* (L.)	Dill	+
Apium graveolens (Mill.)	Celery	+
Daucus carota (L.)	Carrot	+
Fumaria sp.	Fumitory	+
Portulaca oleracea (L.)	Common purslane	+
Rubus fruticosus (agg) - seed	Blackberry	+
Rubus fruticosus (agg) – thorn	Blackberry	+
Stellaria sp.	Chickweed	+
Umbelliferae	Umbellifers	+
Vitis vinifera (L.)	Grape seed	++

Table 7.4. Seashell material.

Scientific Name	Common Name	Quantity
Acanthocardia tuberculata (L.)	Rough cockle	+
Aequipecten opercularis (L.)	Queen scallop	+
Arca noae (L.)	Noah's ark shell	+
Bittium sp. (*tesselatum* (Mts.))	Horn snail	+
Bolinus brandaris (L.)	Purple dye murex	+
Cerastoderma edule (L.) or *glaucum* (Poir.)	Common/edible cockle or lagoon cockle	+
Cerithiidae indet.	Cerith	+
cf. *Cerithium* sp.	Cerith	+
Chamelea gallina (L.)	Striped venus	+
Columbella rustica (L.)	Rustic dove-shell	+
Diodora italica (Def.)	Limpoet	+

The Preliminary Results from a Herculaneum Sewer

Donacilla cornea (Poli)	Corneous wedge clam	++
Donax trunculus (L.)	Truncate *donax*	+
Ensis minor (Che.)	Minor jackknife clam	+
Gibbula albida (Gmel.)	Whitish gibbula	+
Gibbula sp.	Top snail	+
Glycymeris sp.	Bittersweet clam	+
Gregariella cf. *petagnae* (Sca.)	Half-hairy mussel	+
Helicidae	Land snail	++
Hexaplex trunculus (L.)	*Trunculus* murex	+
cf. Muricidae	Murex family	+
Mytilaster cf. *minimus* (Poli)	Mussel	+
cf. *Mytilidae*	Mussel	+
Mytilus galloprovincialis Lam.	Mediterranean mussel	+
Nassarius cf. *costulatus* subspecies *cuvierii* (Pay.)	Dog whelk	+
Nassarius cf. *corniculum* (Olivi)	Horn nassa	+
Ocenebra erinaceus (L.)	Hedgehog murex	+
Ocinebrina edwardsii (Pay.)	Sea snail	+
cf. *Odostomia eulimoides* (Han.)	Pyram	+
Ostrea edulis (L.)	Common/edible oyster	+
Paracentrotus lividus	Stony sea urchin	++
Patella sp.	Limpet	++
Pecten jacobaeus (L.)	Great scallop/pilgrim's scallop	+
Polititapes aureus (Gmel.)	Golden carpet shell	+
Spatangoida	Heart urchin	+
Spondylus gaederopus (L.)	European thorny oyster	+
cf. *Tonna galea* (L.)	Giant tun	+
Turritella communis (Riss.)	Auger shell	+
Venerupis decussata (L.)	Chequered carpet shell	+

the architecture, that the residents were of middle to lower socioeconomic status. The sample findings strengthen this hypothesis. The almost complete absence of imported items suggests that these residents could not often afford such foods. In addition, barring the date seed none of the food items could be classified as luxury goods. Remains of luxury foods such as suckling pigs, wild boar and black pepper have been found at Pompeii, signifying that such items were available in the region (Ciaraldi 2007, 114–115; King 2002, 436–445). While it appears that they could only afford local foods, the fertile nature of the Vesuvian region provided them a diverse and varied diet.

The diversity of items such as shellfish and grains in the sample was somewhat surprising but not unexpected for a coastal town situated near a prime agricultural area. Traditionally, the ancient sources have led modern scholars to believe not only that wheat was a staple crop, but that the Romans preferred it over other grain types (Pliny *HN* 18.62, 18.92–94). However, aside from emmer and einkorn wheat, the sample also contained barley and two varieties of millet. Pliny states that barley is used by the Greeks to make porridge but that the Romans used it only as animal feed (Pliny *HN,* 18.73–75). Although only two barley seeds were found, both were carbonized and their presence in an urban, rather than rural setting, suggests that it was being consumed by humans and not used to feed animals.

When discussing millet Pliny does state that it grows well in the region, but goes on to specifically mention that it is one of the staple grains for those living on the eastern side of the Black Sea (Pliny *HN,* 18.100). While it may have been true that those living off the *frumentatio* in Rome ate only wheat, this does not seem to apply to those living at *Insula Orientalis* II. Millet is the third most common type of edible plant material in the sample. Since it was grown in the region it is not surprising that the inhabitants were using it as a source of food (Pliny *HN,* 18.73–75). The grain variety found in the sample presents a different picture than the statements of ancient authors and it is clear that the people living in *Insula Orientalis* II did not share these prejudices against millet and barley.

In addition to the grain diversity, there were 40 types of shellfish found in the sample (although not all are edible). Interestingly, all the species share two distinct characteristics. They are all small creatures that live in shallow coastal waters (Mojetta 1996, 144–155). These two characteristics provide crucial information about the availability and cost of seafood. Since these animals live in shallow waters it would have been feasible to gather most of them throughout the year. Creatures such as the stony sea urchin and limpet could be collected simply by wading in the shallows, using knifes or sticks to pry them off the rocks. The proximity of Herculaneum to the coast would have made this a quick and easy activity as the sea front was shallow with a depth of only 0.5–0.7 metres (Sigurdsson 2002, 55). As a result, shellfish are a rich source of animal protein that those living in an apartment could frequently afford. The presence of sea urchin in every sample, despite the fact that they were normally considered expensive food items in Roman times, strongly lends support to the idea that certain types of seafood were frequently available at a low cost (Pliny *Ep.* 1.15.1–4, Dalby 2003, 296). The shellfish may have been essential to the diets of the inhabitants since the small sizes of the shells and variety of species suggest that they were not being very selective about their finds. It is possible that they could not afford to be choosy. Larger shellfish would obviously provide more food but may not have been available along the coast and then would have been more expensive.

While the inhabitants who lived above the sewer clearly ate a large variety of foods, it is obvious from the number and frequency of the finds, that some food types were a common and important part of the diet. Eggshell, limpets, wedge clams, sea urchin, fig pips and grape seeds were found in all the stratigraphic levels of both samples (Figure 7.2).

The Preliminary Results from a Herculaneum Sewer

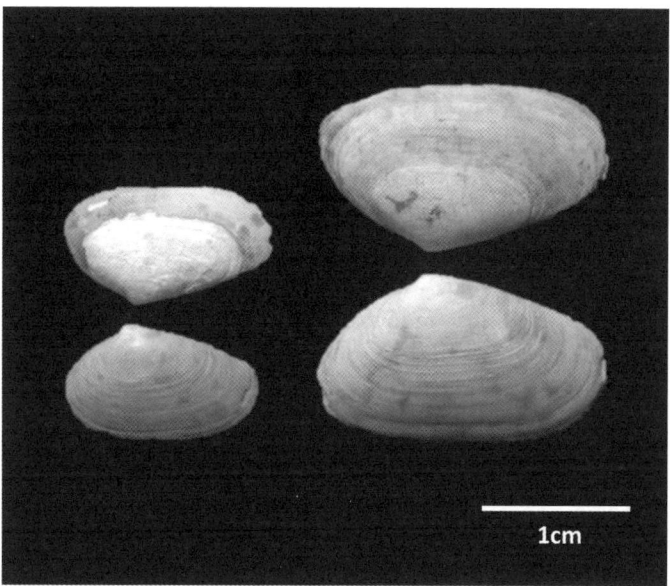

*Figure 7.2: Ancient corneous wedge clams (*Donacilla cornea*) from Quadrant 13–14 (Photo: author).*

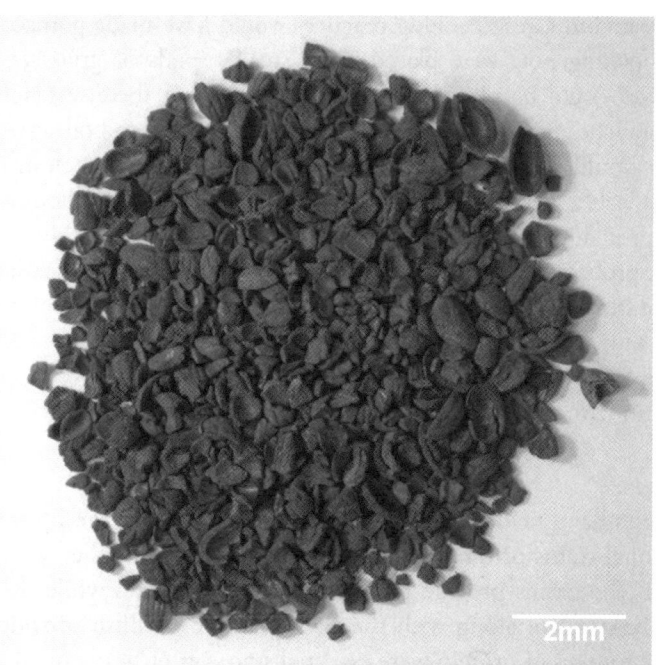

Figure 7.3: Ancient olive stone fragments from Quadrant 3–4. Scale in cm. (Photo: author).

One of the most common non-food items found in the sample is burnt olive stones (Figure 7.3). Although olives were occasionally used for burnt offerings and a few would have been accidentally burnt during food preparation processes, their numbers in the sample suggest that they were used as more than just religious items. Instead, it is likely that these olive stones come from the pressing waste (pomace) generated during olive oil production. After pressing, the olive stones and the remaining paste could have been packed into small cakes and used as cooking fuel (Warnock 2007, 48–51). Pomace gives off huge amounts of energy; one kilogram of pomace is equal to a litre of fuel. In addition, when burnt it gives off little smoke, which would have been beneficial to those living in an upper floor apartment with only windows for ventilation (Brun 2003, 183).

Both the archaeological and literary sources attest to the use of pomace as fuel for cooking and heating. Pliny states that olive stones make the best fire for heating olive oil presses (Pliny *HN* 15.22). In the *Digest*, along with twigs and charcoal, olive stones are described as an alternate source of fuel (*Digest* 32.55). During the Maresha excavations in Israel, 35 carbonized olive stones were found inside a socket in a large subterranean complex dating to the second half of the second century BC. It is believed that the socket worked as a heating installation connected with the olive oil production that took place in the neighbouring rooms (Kloner 2003, 58–59). During the second half of the third century AD, potters in Acharnes near Athens used pomace to heat their kilns (Brun 2003, 184).

These examples suggest that pomace could reach very high temperatures when burned. If it is true that pomace could be used to heat kilns then it could surely boil water. The nature of Roman and Greek cooking practices would have made pomace cakes an ideal fuel source. Cooking pots were placed upon small tripods or grills set on top of the hearth. Charcoal could be placed underneath the pot but there was not enough space using twigs, branches or kindling to make a fire hot enough to boil water. The compact pomace cakes would have easily fitted beneath the pot and their clean burning would have made it a viable fuel source for those living in small spaces without a proper hearth, such as the upper floor apartments at *Insula Orientalis* II. Presumably some sort of fire resistant base, probably a ceramic tile, would need to be placed beneath the pomace so that it did not burn directly on and damage the floor. There are numerous villas in the Vesuvian area with olive oil presses, such as the Villa Pisanella at Boscoreale, Casa di Miri at Gragnano and San Sebastiano (Brun 2004, 13–14). These would have supplied the people of Herculaneum with a local source of pomace.

Nutrition

The two samples have yielded a sufficient amount of evidence for a primary evaluation of the nutritional status of the inhabitants. Firstly, it appears they were eating a well-balanced diet. The grains provide the essential carbohydrates while the legumes such as lentil and broadbean, along with the eggs, fish and shellfish provide the necessary protein. These sources of protein were essential since very few mammal and bird bones were found in the sample, suggesting these people ate little meat. The various fruits and vegetables, such as figs, apples and pears, and celery would have provided the other essential nutrients.

This apparent high seafood, high vegetable protein, low red meat diet is in line with Bisel and Bisel's isotopic studies of the bones from Herculaneum. They analysed the levels of zinc, strontium and calcium in the bones of 139 eruption victims found in beach-front chambers in 1982. The results showed that zinc values were low while the strontium values were high. The authors concluded that the inhabitants of Herculaneum had a diet that was high in seafood and protein-rich vegetables while low in red meat (Bisel and Bisel 2002, 451–458). This is in accordance with the findings of this study.

Therefore, it seems that the human remains and environmental evidence complement one another to a high degree. More importantly, this demonstrates that the collection of food items in the sample are not simply chance finds but instead accurately reflect the larger dietary trends of those living in Herculaneum at the time of the eruption.

In conclusion, the people living in *Insula Orientalis II*, while perhaps not eating expensive or exotic foods, were eating a large range of local foods which provided them with a diet that was diverse, flavourful and nutritious. Further work on the sewer will no doubt expand our knowledge and understanding of diet in Herculaneum, particularly amongst the middle and lower classes.[3]

Notes
1. The pipes in Herculaneum do not show the build up of calcium carbonate that is found in the Serino aqueduct, and instead the water probably came from a spring on the slopes of Vesuvius (Camardo, 2007a).
2. The material farther to the south and the east-west branch had already been excavated by Maiuri in 1949 (Camardo 2008; Maiuri 1958, 467–469).
3. The work presented here was undertaken by the author as part of their Master's thesis.

References
Andrews, J. (March 5, 2012). Insula Orientalis II: Latrine and drain pipes. Pers. comm.
Bisel, S.C. and Bisel, J.F. 2002. 'Health and Nutrition at Herculaneum: An Examination of Human Skeletal Remains', in Jashemski, W. and Meyer, F. (eds.), *The Natural History of Pompeii*, Cambridge, 451–475.
Brun, J.P. 2003. *Le Vin et l'Huile dans la Mediterranée Antique: viticulture, oléicultur et procédés de transformation*, Paris.
Brun, J.P. 2004. *Archaeologie du Vin et l'Huile dans l'Empire Romain*, Paris.
Camardo, D. 2006–2007. *Ercolano: Lo scavo della fogna dell'Insula Orientalis II*. Herculaneum Conservation Project, Unpublished report.
Camardo, D. 2007a. 'Ercolano. La Gestione delle Acque in una Città Romana', *Oebalus: studi sulla Campania nell'Antichità* 2, 167–185.
Camardo, D. 2007b. 'Archaeology and Conservation at Herculaneum: From the Maiuri Campaign to the Herculaneum Conservation Project', *Conservation and Management of Archaeological Sites* 8, 205–214.

Camardo, D. [Email] Message to Dr. Mark Robinson. Accessed 11 March 2009.
Camardo, D. 2008. 'Lo scavo della fogna di Insula Orientalis II' in Guzzo, P.G. and Guidobaldi, M.P. (eds.), *Nuove ricerche archeologiche nell'area vesuviana (scavi 2003–2006): atti del convegno internazionale, Roma, 1–3 febbraio 2007*, Roma, 415–421.
Camardo D., Castaldi, M. and Thompson, J. 2006. 'Water Supply and Drainage in Herculaneum', *Cura aquarum in Ephesus: Proceedings of the Twelfth International Congress on the History of Water Management and Hydraulic Engineering in the Mediterranean Region, Ephesus/Selçuk, Turkey, October 2–10, 2004. (Bulletin antieke beschaving.* Supplement 6), Massachusetts, 183–191.
Casson, L. 1980. 'The role of the state in Rome's grain trade', *Memoirs of the American Academy in Rome* 36, 21–33.
Ciaraldi, M. 2007. *People and plants in ancient Pompeii: a new approach to urbanism from the microscope room: the use of plant resources at Pompeii and in the Pompeian area from the 6th century BC to AD 79*, Specialist Studies on Italy 12, London.
Dalby, A. 2000. *Empire of Pleasures*, New York.
Dalby, A. 2003. *Food in the Ancient World from A to Z*, London.
DeKind, R. 1998. *Houses in Herculaneum: a new view on the town planning and the building of insulae III and IV*, Amsterdam.
Dincauze, D.F. 2000. *Environmental Archaeology*, Cambridge.
Green, F.J. 1979. 'Phosphatic Mineralization of Seeds from Archaeological Sites', *Journal of Archaeological Science* 6, 279–284.
Jansen, G.C.M. 1991. 'Water Systems and Sanitation in the Houses of Herculaneum', *Mededelingen van het Nederlands Instituut te Rome 50*, Netherlands, 145–166.
Jansen, G.C.M. 2000. 'Systems for the Disposal of Waste and Excreta in Roman Cities. The Situation in Pompeii, Herculaneum and Ostia', in Dupré Raventós, X. and Remolà Vallverdú, J.A. (eds.), *Sordes Urbis: la eliminación de residuos en la ciudad romana: actas de la Reunión de Roma, 15–16 de Noviembre de 1996*, Rome, 37–49.
King, A. 2002. 'Mammals: Evidence from Wall Paintings, Sculptures, Mosaics, Faunal Remains, and Ancient Literary Sources', in Jashemski, W. and Meyer, F. (eds.), *The Natural History of Pompeii*, Cambridge, 401–450.
Kloner, A. 2003. *Maresha Excavations Final Report*, Jerusalem.
Maiuri, A. 1948. *Herculaneum*, (6th ed.), Rome.
Maiuri, A. 1958. *Ercolano: i nuovi scavi (1927–1958)*, Roma, Libreria della Stato.
McCobb, L.M.E., Briggs, D.E.G., Evershed, R.P., Hall, A.R. and Hall, R.A. 2001. 'Preservation of Fossil Seeds from a 10th Century AD Cess Pit at Coppergate, York', *Journal of Archaeological Science* 28, 929–940.
Mojetta, A. 1996. *Mediterranean Sea: Guide to the Underwater Life*, London.
Mols, S. 1999. *Wooden Furniture in Herculaneum: Form, Technique and Function*. Vol.2, Amsterdam.
Monteix, N. 2010. *Les lieux de métier: boutiques et ateliers d'Herculanum*, École française de Rome, Rome.
Pesandro, F. and Guidobaldi, M. 2006. *Pompei, Oplontis, Ercolana, Stabiae*, Rome.
Rickman, G. 1980. *The Corn Supply of Ancient Rome*, Oxford.
Robinson, M., Fulford, N. and Tootell, K. 2006. 'The Macroscopic Plant Remains', in Fulford, M., Clarke, A. and Eckardt, H. (eds.), *Life and Labour in Late Roman Silchester: Excavations in Insula IX since 1997* (Britannia Monograph Series No. 22), London, 206–218.
Robinson, M. 2007a. (Unpublished report). *The Archaeological Potential of the Herculaneum Sewer*.
Robinson, M. 2007b. (Unpublished report). *Preliminary Report on the Processing of Samples from Herculaneum Cardo V Fogna*.
Sigurdsson H. and Carey, S. 2002. 'The Eruption of Vesuvius in AD 79', in Jashemski, W. and Meyer, F. (eds.), *The Natural History of Pompeii*, Cambridge, 37–64.
Wallace-Hadrill, A. 1994. *Houses and Society in Pompeii and Herculaneum*, Princeton.
Warnock, P. 2007. *Identification of ancient olive oil processing methods based on olive remains*, Oxford.

The 1270 Durrës Earthquake Victims from the Roman Amphitheatre Excavations: a Global Palaeonutritional Study of an Anthropological and Archaeological Sample

Sara Santoro, Antonietta Buglione, Giovanni De Venuto, Paola Iacumin, Barbara Sassi, and Loretana Salvadei

University of Chieti-Pescara (Santoro), University of Foggia (Buglione, De Venuto), University of Parma (Iacumin, Sassi), Museo Etnografico Pigorini, Rome (Salvadei)

Introduction (by Sara Santoro)

The Durrës amphitheatre is one of the largest in the Balkan Peninsula and was probably built by the emperor Trajan (98–118 AD), who promoted urban growth in association with the second Dacian war. The monument likely functioned as an amphitheatre until the fourth century AD, when an important seismic event (*c*. 346 AD) appears to have contributed to its abandonment. In the Byzantine period (fifth–sixth centuries) walls were built close to, and abutted the external façade of, the amphitheatre. From at least the eighth century the arena and the galleries of the amphitheatre functioned as a necropolis and were also used as housing. The presence of chapels with apses, built in the *fornices* of the amphitheatre and decorated with paintings and mosaics, attests to re-use of the monument for Christian worship in the sixth–ninth centuries.

The amphitheatre is located in the south-west of the ancient city and south-east of the hill that dominates the town. The amphitheatre, perhaps still visible at the beginning of the sixth century, disappeared in the following centuries, buried by the soil which collapsed from the hill against which it was constructed, and probably also due to the landslides triggered by the frequent seismic events in the area. On the hill slope, houses were built both in the Turkish era and after the Second World War, removing all visible traces of the amphitheatre.

Parts of the arena, cavea and the galleries were re-discovered during excavations undertaken since 1966, carried out by the Albanian archaeologist Vangjel Toçi. These excavations were never extended to the whole amphitheatre area. Excavation resumed in 2003 under the Durrës Project, an International Cooperation Agreement for the safeguard of the archaeological heritage of Durrës, signed between Parma University, the United Nations Office for Project Service (UNOPS), the Archaeological Museum of Durrës, the Archaeological Institute of the Academy of Sciences, the Durrës Municipality and the Culture Monument Institute of the Albanian Ministry for Culture, Youth and Sports. In 2004 excavations were undertaken in the southern part of the amphitheatre by archaeologists from the University of Parma, directed by Prof. Sara Santoro, with the support of the Italian Ministry for Foreign Affairs (MAE-DGPCC-uff.V), the Italian Archaeological Mission and the Cultural Cooperation Project of Durrës Urban Archaeological Park, in collaboration with the Durrës Department of Archaeology, directed by Prof. Afrim Hoti, with the obvious importance of the Roman monument for the city of Durrës leading to it immediately becoming one of the key elements of the future urban archaeological park (Santoro 2004; Hoti et al. 2003). A multidisciplinary approach has been taken with the research project, with specialists in geophysical prospection, archaeometry and architecture all contributing to the archaeological study, architectural survey and a restoration project.

The aim of this project was to elucidate the stratigraphic context from which the recovered skeletal and faunal remains originated. This can be divided into two main sections. The first section consists of the galleries I–IX of the amphitheatre, and particularly gallery VII, where a small portion of the largest necropolis lies inside the city walls occupying the amphitheatre between eighth and tenth centuries (Gutteridge et al. 2001). The second section is composed of a building (rooms A–G) and an open space facing west (area B/C3) which occupied this part of the amphitheatre from the first half of the twelfth century: from this area, both inside and outside the building, come the remains of the supposed victims of the earthquake and tsunami that struck Durrës one night in March 1270 (Guidoboni and Comastri 2005).

The archaeology of the site *(by Barbara Sassi)*
The galleries of the amphitheatre
In the nine galleries investigated in the southern area of the amphitheatre (Figure 8.1), the excavated layers provide evidence for a series of living spaces occupied from the twelfth–fourteenth centuries. The deposits consist of debris from the 1270 earthwork, including large fragments from the collapsed vaults and cement floor of the amphitheatre. Other layers, including occupation deposits, date from the twelfth–thirteenth centuries. Under the 'ruins' of the earthquake, the remains of at least three individuals have been recovered (two males aged 30–40 and a female aged 40–50). These and other remains are interpreted as victims crushed by the collapsing amphitheatre whose bones became disarticulated by the settling of the collapsed rocks and the later levelling of the area. This area of the amphitheatre appears to have been densely populated in 1270.

An occupation deposit (SU 662) rich in coarse pottery and amphorae (twelfth century) covered and damaged a series of inhumations which partially leant against the stairs of gallery n.7. Human bones of at least five individuals were recovered. Underneath, tombs 1, 2, 3 and 5, located in roofing-tile coffins, were placed approximately on an east-west alignment with the skulls to the west, while tomb 4 was aligned north-south, close to the eastern wall of the gallery.

The skeletal material was fragmentary and incomplete except in three cases (tomb 1 SU 661: a male aged over 50; tomb 2 SU 698: a female aged 30–40 and tomb 4 SU 724: a possible female aged 2–3 months). In both tomb 3 and 5 there were at least two

The 1270 Durrës Earthquake Victims

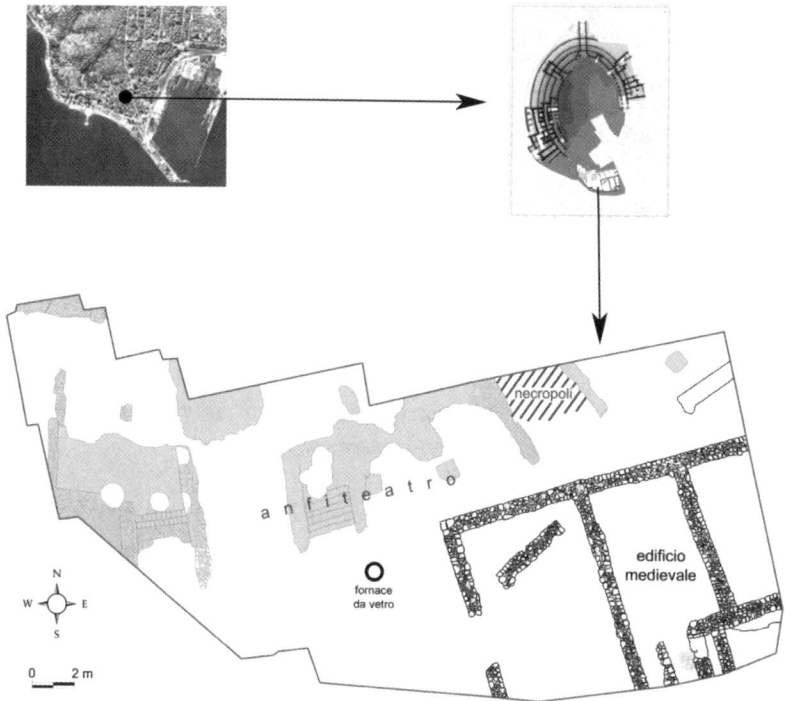

Figure 8.1. The Roman amphitheatre (anfiteatro) in Dürres. To the north-east is a necropolis, to the south a glass kiln and to the east a medieval building.

individuals whose sex could not be determined (tomb 3a SU 721: age about 1 year; tomb 3b SU 722: age about 2 years; tomb 5a SU 727: age 2–3 months and tomb 5b SU 727: age about 6 months). None of the tombs contained objects. The presence of multiple tombs, containing several skeletons in succession, may explain the use of a tomb by the same family over a protracted period (Ivison 1996).

The medieval building
In the south-eastern area of the excavation a building with substantial walls was partially revealed and in 2007 its wider extent was determined through geophysical survey. The building consists of multiple phases of beaten earth floors and appears to have been occupied from the thirteenth century to the present day. Deposits associated with the 1270 earthquake are clearly differentiated from the structural phases of reconstruction (shown in the beaten floors SU 606–652–651 and in the construction of partition walls) and the levelling of the ruins from the late thirteenth to the fifteenth century. In rooms A–C (Figure 8.2) a crumbled layer (SU 682), containing monochrome, coarse and tin-glazed (decorated with spirals) pottery and amphorae sherds of thirteenth-century date, was excavated beneath a later dump. This layer covered a poorly preserved terracotta

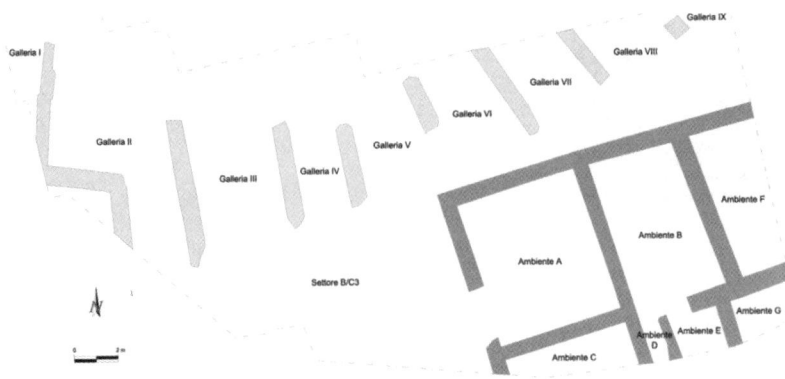

Figure 8.2. Map of archaeological features (galleria) *in the southern part of the Dürres amphitheatre (area B). To the south you can see several rooms.*

tiled floor (SU 682). The stratigraphic sequence in Rooms B and E is similar to that of rooms A–C, with the same beaten floors and occupation layers being present at the same levels.

The skeletal remains of four individuals, in a good state of preservation, were recovered from rooms A–C. These were incorporated in deposit SU 658 and over the floor layer SU 682. In the middle of the area, two adults; a female aged 30 (victim 2) and a male aged older than 50 (victim 3) were oriented north-south (skull to the south). A male child of 2–3 years of age (victim 4) lay at the feet of the male. To the south lay a female child aged 7–8 years of age (victim 1). No finds were associated with the bodies, except for a tight iron collar which was around the neck of the male adult. The unusual and irregular position of the bodies (victim 1 fallen on her back with the right knee against the breast; victim 2 with a phalanx in the nasal septum) supports the suggestion that these are not typical inhumations. The absence of other possible graves, the stratigraphic position of the bodies, their late thirteenth-century date and their presence in a living space all support the assumption that they are victims of the earthquake of 1270, possibly a family who did not manage to escape outside, being choked and crushed to death by the debris.

Beneath the deposits associated with the rebuilding activity at the end of the thirteenth and beginning of the fourteenth centuries (SU 651), excavation revealed a complex deposit comprising a collapsed tile roof, which showed evidence of burning (SU 665). Beneath the collapsed tiles, the beams and rafters (SU 666) have been recovered. Analysis of the charcoal demonstrated the beam to be of elm/Ulmus and the rafters of southern ash/Fraxinus (Marchesini et al. n.d.). The wooden elements are of varying diameters, suggesting a sloping roof with a main girder, orientated north-south. The collapsed elements were situated on a beaten floor (SU 714=733), from which pottery of thirteenth-century date (monochrome and tin-glazed pottery, a fragment of metallic ware and amphorae) were recovered. This appears to be a closed context, created by a sudden event, probably the earthquake of 1270. Further evidence of the earthquake is provided by small deposits present in room B/C3, a small open space outside of the building, where a thick layer of levelled ruins (SU 265) was present beneath post-earthquake reconstruction deposits.

The construction techniques and stratigraphic sequence show that some walls survived the earthquake, whilst others were rebuilt following the 1270 earthquake and during the Ottoman period (fifteenth–sixteenth centuries). The presence of beaten and tiled floors of thirteenth-century dates, fireplaces and domestic material culture suggest that the buildings functioned as living spaces, and the low quality of the later walls suggests that the later occupation was of relatively low socio-economic status, although it is possible that more extravagant features were removed during later reconstruction. The foundations of the walls date to the early twelfth century, with further evidence of this pre-earthquake phase having been removed by the earthquake of 1270. The building was rebuilt on a plainimetric plan, with large spaces being sub-divided. Occupation continued into the sixteenth century and remained to be partially utilized into the modern period, as shown in data collected during the surveys of 2005–2006 (Santoro, Hoti and Sassi 2008).

The anthropological analysis *(by Loretana Salvadei)*

The anthropological study presented here relates to the four individuals who are interpreted as victims of the 1270 earthquake (Table 8.1). These consist of two adults (victims 2 and 3) and two children (victims 1 and 4). As detailed above, these were found beneath debris associated with the 1270 earthquake and the bones are well-preserved. A further three victims, crushed by the falling blocks, were found outside of the palace (victim 5; victim SU 485 CN; victim SU 485 AFL) (Ferembach et al. 1977–79).

Analysis of tooth pathology, caries, dental abcesses and tooth loss, was undertaken as these provide the most direct indicators of diet. Most dental-alveolar pathologies derive from the interaction between dietetic factors (fibrous structure and chemical composition of consumed food) and bacterial flora, usually found in dental plaque that builds up on teeth. When a diet consists mainly of carbohydrates, the organic acids deriving from their bacterial fermentation act on the enamel or cementum causing decalcification and, consequently, tooth decay (Larsen 1997). The infection which develops around the periapical tissue may evolve into an abscess and lead to possible tooth loss. The excessive consumption of carbohydrates is certainly one of the main causes of dental caries, although other factors, such as hereditary predisposition and oral hygiene, should be taken into account. Apart from determining the type of diet, the survey aimed to identify whether the victims were of different socio-economic status, based on their diet.

In the sample examined, the incidence of caries on the anterior teeth confirms the common consumption of carbohydrates associated with poor tooth care. Moreover, the three affected adults showed several lesions (victim 2, victim 3, victim CN). A larger

The 1270 Durrës Earthquake Victims

Table 8.1. Gender and age list of earthquake victims (* bone's fragments from 'exterior victims' not referable to three individuals).

Individuals	Gender	Age
Interior victims:		
victim 1 SU 616	F?	7–8 years
victim 2 SU 642	F	c. 30 years
victim 3 SU 641	M	50+ years
victim 4	M	2–3 years
Exterior victims:		
Victim 5	M	30–40 years
SU 485 CN	M	30–40 years
SU 485 AFL	F	40–50 years
* SU 485 B	?	Adult
* SU 485 D	?	Adult
* SU 485 E	?	Adult
* SU 485 M	?	Adult

number of caries were present in the contact area between two teeth, indicating that the remains of food in interdental space may have affected the aetiology of lesions. Victim 3 shows abscesses, perforations of the alveolar surface, as well as tooth loss, which is identifiable by the process of reabsorption of the alveolar bone (Brothwell 1981). The posterior teeth are the most damaged since they are involved in the chewing process; this confirms the role of food remains and the consequent acid fermentation as cariogenic factors. A further indication of vegetarian diet comes from three cases of tooth decay on the deciduous molars of victim 1 (7–8 years), due to dietary factors rather than a lack of calcification. On the other side, the enamel hypoplasia visible on the crowns seems to be compatible with possible food deficiencies (Goodman et al. 1980; Goodman and Rose 1991).

The presence of *cribra orbitalia*, a condition characterized by clusters of small openings in the portions of the orbital plate of the frontal bone, was found in three of the seven analysed individuals (victim 2, victim 4, victim 5). This suggests that severe anaemia was widespread. The absence of additional skeletal deformities suggests that this relates to an iron-deficient, cereal diet and poor hygienic conditions, rather than conditions such as rickets, scurvy or hereditary anaemia (El-Najjar 1976; Stuart-Macadam 1989).

Overall the results suggest poor sanitary conditions and diet. The tooth pathology suggests a vegetable-rich diet whilst the presence of *cribra orbitalia* suggests a diet deficient in iron. The results could suggest that the internal group are of a different social class to those found on the exterior of the buildings, although such a conclusion cannot be confirmed on the anthropological analysis alone.

The isotopic analysis *(by Paola Iacumin)*

Over the last thirty years, the application of isotopic analysis in archaeology has developed greatly, with oxygen, carbon and nitrogen isotopes being used to reconstruct past landscapes, economies and diets, as well as the movements of groups or single individuals within a region, and sometimes ancient rituals. Stable isotopes of the above listed elements are present in various parts of an organism, and analysis of these allows us to document the diverse nutritional contributions made by food and water. This information is fixed during the course of an organism's life in both the organic (for example, collagen, which represents the organic components of bones and teeth) and inorganic tissues (for example, bone and tooth apatite) (Ambrose 1993; DeNiro and Epstein 1978; Longinelli 1984). Put simply, such evidence gives credence to the expression: 'You are what you eat'.

Carbon and nitrogen have two stable isotopes each, ^{12}C, ^{13}C and ^{14}N, ^{15}N, respectively. Oxygen has three, ^{16}O, ^{17}O and ^{18}O, but normally, it is the first and second isotopes that are measured, being the most abundant.

The isotopic relationship is generally reported in parts per thousand (‰), relative to an international standard, with the isotopic value noted using the definition 'δ'.

$$\delta = (R_{sample}/R_{standard} - 1) * 1000 \text{ where } R = {}^{13}C/{}^{12}C, \text{ or } R = {}^{15}N/{}^{14}N, \text{ or } R = {}^{18}O/{}^{16}O.$$

Oxygen

The study of oxygen isotopes in the phosphate of fossilized mammal bone and tooth apatite has led to the reconstruction of paleo-climatic conditions for at least the last million years. Such analysis depends on the direct relationship existing between the isotope composition of phosphate ($\delta^{18}O_p$) and the mean isotope composition of meteoric water ($\delta^{18}O_w$) in the area where the organism lived. This relationship, best described in a first-order equation, is typical for every species of every mammal, being also a function of the biological characteristics of every group, and the differences with their own metabolic processes (Longinelli 1984). On the basis of such equations, and of the isotopic measurements of oxygen in phosphate, it is therefore possible to calculate the average isotopic relationship of the water in a given environment. Since water of meteoric origin is used by different individuals, its isotopic value is a function of the median annual temperature of the soil, and depending on the case, the level of humidity, and can therefore provide information on the paleo-climatic and paleo-environmental conditions (Longinelli 1995).

The carbonate in the bone and tooth apatite is another source of oxygen that is measured isotopically. Recent studies have proven that the oxygen in this carbonate is in equilibrium with phosphate oxygen, since each develop in equilibrium with oxygen found in the water of the body (Iacumin et al. 1996). This measurement, beyond providing the same 'climatic' information as phosphate, is much more useful as a control of the reliability of isotopic values, above all in the cases of finds preserved in particularly humid, hot, and/or relatively 'old' (>Pleistocene) environments, that were able to be subjected to alternation due to diagenetic processes.

Carbon and nitrogen

Most recently, another research technique has been fine-tuned, which is based on the isotopic composition of carbon ($\delta^{13}C_{col}$) and nitrogen ($\delta^{15}N$) in collagen and carbonate apatite ($\delta^{13}C_{carb}$). This can lead to the reconstruction of eating habits, and therefore provide important information related to the environment. For example, the isotope ratio of carbon in the collagen and in the apatite allows us to distinguish a diet based on plants with C_3 photosynthetic cycle (trees and plants typical of temperate and cold environment) (mean value of $\delta^{13}C = -26.5‰$) from a diet based on plants with C_4 photosynthetic cycle (maize, millet) (mean value of $\delta^{13}C = -12.5‰$). Furthermore, the isotope ratio of collagen carbon represents the protein fraction of the diet while the isotope ratio of apatite carbon represents the average value of the diet. The isotope ratio of nitrogen gives information on the trophic level of the animals, being related to the protein consumption in the diet. With regard to human beings, this ratio allows one to distinguish a diet based on terrestrial products from one based on sea or fresh-water resources (Chisholm et al. 1982; Schoeninger and DeNiro 1984). Additionally, to have at one's disposal both bone and teeth fragments from the same individual, yields information on the nomadic or sedentary character of a whole population or a single individual.

Results

Nine individuals were studied, of which three came from early medieval burials, four were considered victims of the 1273 earthquake and found in a medieval building, while two more were likely victims of the same earthquake, but buried under the collapse of the amphitheatre, external to the building. Five individuals had their rib, and their first and their third molars measured; two individuals had just the rib and the first molar measured; for one, their first and third molars, and for another just the rib. The isotopic composition of oxygen and carbon ($\delta^{18}O_{carb}$), of carbonate, of the isotope composition of carbon ($\delta^{13}C_{coll}$) and of nitrogen ($\delta^{15}N_{coll}$) in collagen were measured for all skeletal remains in this sample.

The analysis of carbon and nitrogen reveals a small difference between the early medieval skeletons and the victims of the earthquake, with less negative values ($\delta^{13}C_{carb}$, $\delta^{13}C_{coll}$) and more positive ($\delta^{15}N_{coll}$) for the first group (see Table 8.2 and Figures 8.2–8.3). This might point to a small contribution made by C_4 plants in the early medieval diet, not seen in the victims of the earthquake except for the individual V3– SU 641 during the first years of their life. The analysis reveals that the diet of all the individuals was based on terrestrial resources.

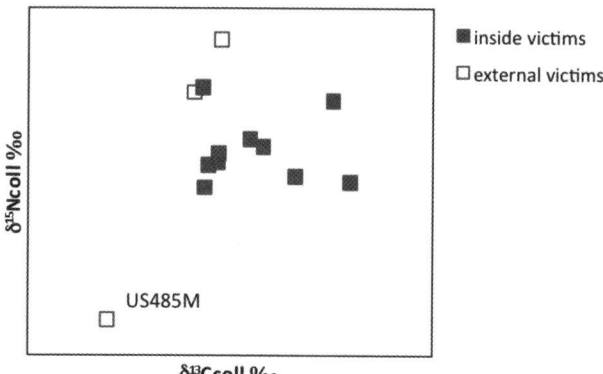

Figure 8.3: Nitrogen and carbon isotope composition of collagen. The "vegetarian" individual has lower nitrogen values than the others.

Table 8.2. Isotopic ratios (‰) of carbon and oxygen in the carbonate apatite, isotope composition of carbon and nitrogen in the collagen and C/N ratio.

	sex/age (years)	$\delta^{13}C_{carb}$	$\delta^{18}O_{carb}$	$\delta^{13}C_{coll}$	$\delta^{15}N_{coll}$	C/N
Inside amphitheatre						
V1-SU 616 rib	F? 7-8	-12.8	30.2	-19.3	7.5	3.2
V1-SU 616 C1 left	F? 7-8	-13.2	30.3	-19.2	7.8	3.2
V1-SU 616 M1 left	F? 7-8	-13.7	30.2	-18.7	8.2	3.1
V2-SU 642 rib	F c.30	-13.1	29.5	-19.4	6.9	3.1
V2-SU 642 M1 right	F c.30	-13.5	30.6	-18.5	8.0	3.2
V2-SU 642 M3 left	F c.30	-12.1	29.8	-18.0	7.2	3.2
V3-SU 641 rib	M 50+	-13.5	29.2	-19.2	7.6	3.0
V3-SU 641 M1 right	M 50+	-12.1	31.1	-17.5	9.3	3.3
V3-SU 641 M3 right	M 50+	-10.5	28.3	-17.2	7.0	3.2
V4 rib	M 2-3	-13.5	29.6	-19.4	9.7	3.1
V4 M1 left	M 2-3	-13.3	29.6	-18.8		
average		-12.8	29.9	-18.7	7.9	3.2
Outside amphitheatre						
SU 485 C M1 left	M 30-40	-13.6	27.5	-19.1	11.1	3.3
SU 485 C M3 left	M 30-40	-13.4	26.5	-19.5	9.6	3.2
SU 485 M rib	F 40-50	-10.3	30.1	-20.8	3.0	3.1

Among the victims of the earthquake found outside the building, the individual SU 485-find M differs from the others, having a particularly low value of carbon and nitrogen (see Table 8.2 and Figure 8.2), perhaps indicating a diet very low in animal proteins. The other individual found outside the building (SU 485-find C) differs from all the other skeletons, having lower values of oxygen (Table 8.2 and Figure 8.3), indicating, probably, a different place of origin with respect to the other individuals.

The analysis does not reveal differences between the sexes, although the sample size is small. The first molar generally shows an enrichment in heavy oxygen and nitrogen compared with the third molar and the skeletal bone for the same individual, showing the effect of diet on Molar 1 (Table 8.1 and Figure 8.1). The first molar, in fact, begins to mineralize at birth. The two juvenile skeletons, both children aged 2–3 years, show enrichment in heavy nitrogen in the bones compared with the older individuals, an effect of breastfeeding.

The faunal sample *(by Antonietta Buglione)*
Quantitative data
This discussion is a preliminary report on the thirteenth–fifteenth century faunal remains from the site. The assemblage consists of 1488 identifiable fragments, representing 240 individuals (Figure 8.4). The bones are generally well-preserved and it is possible to distinguish some natural taphonomic indicators (such as burning and gnawing) and anthropogenic indicators (such as slaughtering and butchering marks).

Sheep/goat are the most abundant species present (54.5%, representing 43.5% of the minimum number of individuals). Pigs were the second most common species. Other domestic animals (dogs, cats and horses) were present, but did not feature in human diet. The low quantity of dog, cat and rodent bones and the scarce presence of gnawing marks on the bones suggest that waste was regularly disposed of and not allowed to linger on the surface. The few poultry remains suggest a negligible subsistence economy.

Wild animals are not frequent in the assemblage. Some roe deer, deer, wild boar, hare and bird bones are present. It is worth noting the presence of two aurochs' (*Bos primigenius*) bones, a fragment of proximal metatarsus (Bp: 68 mm) and a fragment of distal femur (Bd: 120 mm) (dimensions after Von den Driesch 1976). The remains of marine species, including molluscs such as *Cardium* and *Murex,* are rare.

Mortality and sex determination
Following Payne (1973), the sheep/goat cull pattern was examined, observing 72 mandibles and single teeth (Figure 8.5). Sheep/goat were bred for meat and wool production and the animals are mostly mature, having been killed around the age of 4 years. The low quantity of young individuals suggests that there was a negligible use of these animals for milk and dairy products. The ratio between sheep and goats appears to favour sheep, with young ones prevailing with 65% of 37 bones (distinguished after Böessneck et al. 1964).

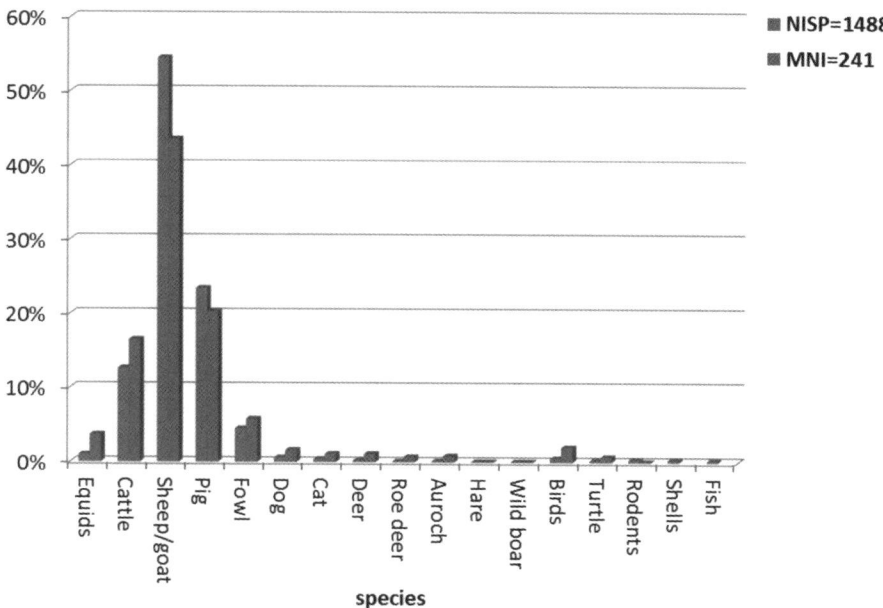

Figure 8.4. The medieval animal bone samples according NISP (Number of Identified Specimen) and MNI (Minimum Number of Individuals).

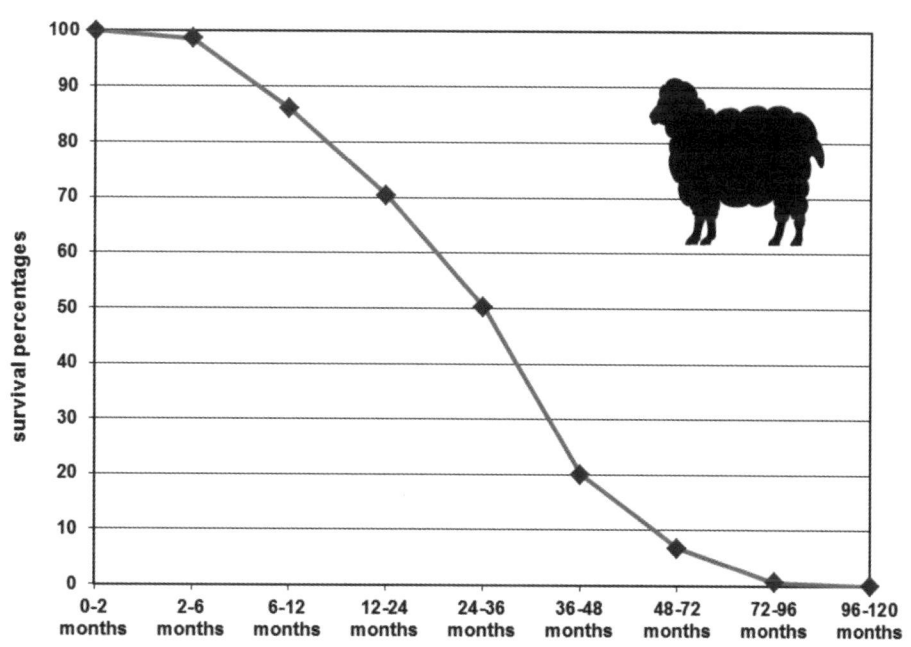

Figure 8.5: The survival curve for sheep/goat.

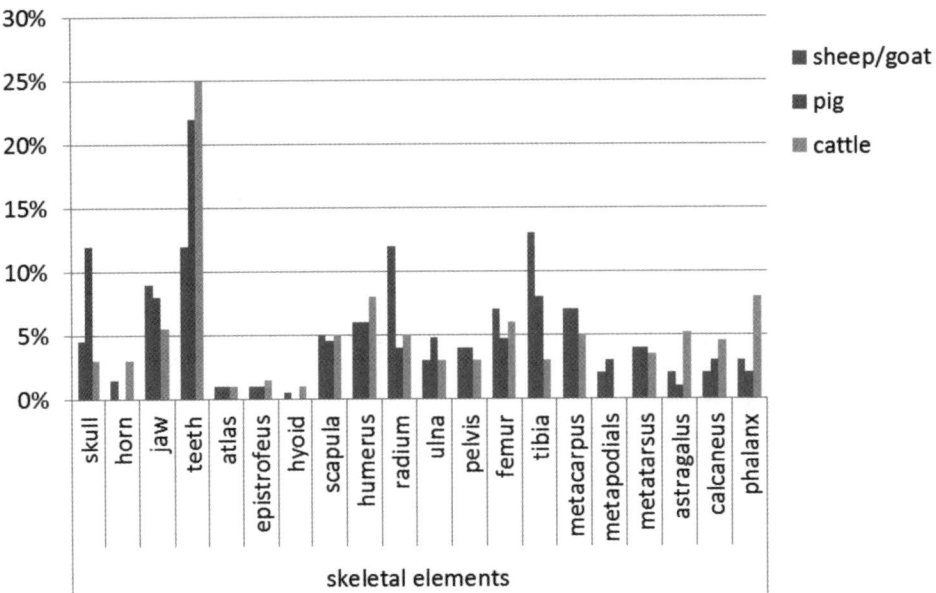

Figure 8.6: The anatomical distribution for cattle, pig and sheep/goats.

The pigs were butchered at the age of two, the optimum time to kill them for good meat and fat, when balanced against the cost of their upkeep (after Bull and Payne 1982). The intensive breeding of these animals is confirmed by the proportion of young individuals (19.2%) for the supply of fresh meat, compared with 34.6% of the assemblage comprising old animals kept for reproduction. This breeding pattern is also shown in the sex distribution; amongst 47 pig bones analysed 85.1% belong to boar. Sows were probably killed less frequently, when they were old and no longer useful for reproduction. Cattle account for a low proportion of the assemblage and were kept principally for traction, as few individuals were killed before the age of three, probably to obtain meat.

Anatomical distribution
The lower and upper limbs of sheep/goat, the parts which are richest in meat, are most abundant in the assemblage (see Figure 8.6). The extremities, such as phalanxes and metapodials, are comparatively rare, since they were discarded during butchery. The high presence of teeth is related to preferential preservation compared with the other anatomical elements and should be contrasted against the low quantity of skulls and skull fragments. Comparatively high quantities of pig and cattle teeth are present.

Some considerations *(by Giovanni De Venuto)*

These data suggest a prevalence of domestic animals in the human diet, with sheep/goats being the most important resource. The mortality pattern shows that their breeding was intended for meat supply. As the anatomical distribution demonstrated, the parts of the animal rich in meat, such as hindlimb and forelimb, were above all present in the *palatium*. The animals were probably bred in the surrounding territory of the city and, after butchering, were exchanged in the urban markets. The importance of the meat supply is confirmed by the pig data, which show evidence of an intensive breeding programme. Unlike sheep and goats, pigs were probably kept around the area of *palatium*.

Wild animals and fish were only minor elements of diet. Aurochs is not frequently present in European medieval faunal assemblages (some examples are in Bartosiewicz 1997; Kyselý 2005) but it often appears in some pre-Roman and Roman assemblages from southern Italy (Farello 1995, 377); it disappeared in the seventeenth century (1627) in Poland (Pyle 1994). The hunting of these animals reveals the hunting skills of higher status individuals. The wild faunal assemblage suggests a natural habitat composed of forests and surrounding open lands for pasture, close to the medieval town.

The data from Durrës can be compared with Stari Bar, an abandoned town in the south-western region of Montenegro. The study by Pluskowski and Seetah (2006) shows sheep/goats to be the most widely exploited animals from the end of the thirteenth to the sixteenth centuries. Here, the representation of anatomical elements is different. There are a high proportion of mandible fragments and limb bones, probably suggesting that sheep were brought into the settlement on the hoof, slaughtered on site and elements of their carcasses redistributed for culinary and industrial uses. A high prevalence of juvenile animals suggests exploitation of animals for milk and dairy products. Unlike the Durrës context, the second most represented species were cattle, killed when they were old.

The zooarchaeological analysis of the Durrës assemblage reveals that the medieval diet was not protein poor. This data contrasts with the results of the anthropological analysis of the 1270 earthquake victims. Probably their presence, inside the *palatium* rooms, was temporary: the slave collar at the neck of the male victim could represent an interpretative key, demonstrating that the faunal remains relate to a different social group to those represented by the human remains from the site.

References

Ambrose, S.H. 1993. 'Isotopic analysis of paleodiets: Methodological and interpretive considerations', in Sandford, K. (ed.), *Investigations of Ancient Human Tissue, Chemical Analyses in Anthropology*, Langhorne, 59–130.

Bartosiewicz, L. 1997. 'A horn worth blowing? A stray find of aurochs from Hungary', *Antiquity* 71, 1007–10.

Böessneck, J., Müller, H.-H. and Teichert, M. 1964. 'Osteologische Unterscheidungsmerkmale zwischen Schaft (*Ovis aries* Linne) und Ziege (*Capra hircus* Linne)', *Kühn-Archiv* 78, H.1–2.

Brothwell, D.R. 1981. *Digging up bones*, Oxford.

Bull, G. and Payne, S. 1982. 'Tooth eruption and epiphisial fusion in pigs and wild boar' in Wilson, B., Grigson, S. and Payne, S. (eds.), *Ageing and sexing animal bones from archeological sites*, BAR British Series 109, Oxford, 55–81.

Chisholm, B.S., Nelson, D.E. and Schwarcz, H.P. 1982. 'Stable carbon isotope ratios as a measure of marine versus terrestrial protein in ancient diets', *Science* 216, 1131–1132.

El-Najjar, M.Y. 1976. 'Maize, malaria and the anemias in the pre-Columbian New World', *Yearbook of Physical Anthropology* 20, 329–337.

DeNiro, M.J. and Epstein, S. 1978. 'Influence of diet on the distribution of carbon isotopes in animals', *Geochimica et Cosmochimica Acta* 42, 495–506.

Farello, P. 1995. 'Diffusione dell'uro in Emilia Romagan dal Neolitico all'età del Ferro', *Atti del 1° Convegno nazionale di archeozoologia (Rovigo 1993), Padusa Quaderni*, 1, Stanghella, 377–379.

Ferembach, D., Schwidetzky, I. and Stloukal, M. 1977–79. 'Raccomandazioni per la determinazione dell'età e del sesso sullo scheletro', *Rivista di Antropologia* 60, 5–51.

Goodman, A.H., Armelagos, G.J. and Rose, J.C. 1980. 'Enamel hypoplasia as indicators of stress in three prehistoric populations from Illinois', *Human Biology* 52, 515–528.

Goodman, A.H. and Rose, J.C. 1991. 'Dental enamel hypoplasias as indicators of nutritional status', in Kelley, M.A. and Larsen, C.S. (eds.), *Advances in Dental Anthropology*, New York, 279–293.

Guidoboni, E. and Comastri, A. (eds.). 2005. *Catalogue of earthquakes and tsunamis in the mediterranea area from the 11th to the 15th century*, Istituto Nazionale di Geofisica e Vulcanologia, Bologna, 279–283.

Gutteridge, A., Hoti, A. and Hurst, A.R. 2001. 'The walled town of Dyrrachium (Durrës): settlements and dynamics', *Journal of Roman Archaeology* 14(1), 391–410.

Hoti, A., Metalla, E. and Shehi, E. 2003. 'Recentissimi scavi archeologici a Durrës 2001–2003', in Santoro, S. and Buora, M. (eds.), *Strumenti per la salvaguardia del patrimonio archeologico: carte del rischio e catalogazione informatizzata – Alte tecnologie applicate all'archeologia di Durrës*, Antichità Altoadriatiche, LVIII, 401–435.

Iacumin, P., Bocherens, H., Mariotti, A. and Longinelli, A. 1996. 'Oxygen isotope analyses of co-existing carbonate and phosphate in biogenic apatite: a way to monitor diagenetic alteration of bone phosphate?' *Earth and Planetary Science Letters* 142, 1–6.

Ivison, E.A. 1996. 'Burial and Urbanism at Late Antique and Early Byzantine Corinth (c.AD 400–700)', in Christie, N. and Loseby, S.T. (eds.), *Towns in Transition. Urban Evolution in late Antiquity and the Early Middle Ages*, Guildford, 99–112.

Kyselý, R. 2005. 'Archeologické doklady divok'ych savců na území ČR v období od neolitu po novověk' [Archaeological evidence of wild mammals in the Czech Republic from the Neolithic to Modern times] *Lynx* 36, 55–101.

Larsen, C.S. 1997. *Bioarchaeology*, Cambridge.

Longinelli, A. 1984. 'Oxygen isotopes in mammal bone phosphate: a new tool for paleohydrological and paleoclimatological research?' *Geochimica et Cosmochimica Acta*, 48, 385–390.

Longinelli, A. 1995. 'Stable isotope ratios in phosphate from mammal bone and tooth as climatic indicators', in Frenzel, B. (ed.), *Proceedings of the ESF Workshop, Bern 1993*, Palaeoklimaforschung Bd 15, Special Issue, 57–70.

Marchesini, M., Martelli, S. and Rizzoli, E. n.d. '*Risultati delle indagini antracologiche sui reperti rinvenuti nell'anfiteatro di Durrës (Durazzo, Albania)*', internal report.

Payne, S. 1973. 'Kill-off patterns in sheep and goats: the mandibles from Aşvan Kale', *Anatolian Studies* 23, 281–303.

Pluskowski, A. and Seetah, K. 2006. 'The animal bones from the 2004 excavation at Stari Bar, Montenegro', in Gelichi, S. (ed.), *The archaeology of an abandoned town,* Firenze, 97–11.

Pyle, C.M. 1994. 'Some late sixteenth-century depictions of the aurochs (*Bos primigenius* Bojanus, extinct 1627): new evidence from Vatican MS Urb. lat. 276', *Archives of Natural History* 21, 275–288.

Schoeninger, M.J. and De Niro, M.J. 1984. 'Nitrogen and carbon isotopic composition of bone-collagen from marine and terrestrial animals', *Geochimica et Cosmochimica Acta* 48, 625–639.

Santoro, S. 2004. 'Il Progetto Pilota 'Progettazione e realizzazione del Parco Archeologico Urbano di Durrës (Albania), Università di Parma e Ministero degli Affari Esteri DGPCC Uff. V – Settore Archeologia 2004', in Buora, M. and Santoro, S. (eds.), '*Progetto Durrës. Strumenti della salvaguardia del patrimonio culturale: carta del rischio archeologico e catalogazione informatizzata. Esempi italiani ed applicabilità in Albania*' (Atti del secondo incontro scientifico, Parma-Udine 27–29 marzo 2003), and in Buora, M. and Santoro, S. (eds.), '*Alte tecnologie applicate all'archeologia di Durrës*' (Atti del terzo incontro scientifico, Durrës 22 giugno 2004), *Antichità Altoadriatiche LVIII*, 429–437.

Santoro, S., Hoti, A. and Sassi, B. (eds.). 2008. 'L'anfiteatro di Durazzo. Studi e scavi 2004–2005', *ASAtene, LXXXIII,* 2004, s. III-4, Tomo 2, 717–808.

Stuart-Macadam, P.L. 1989. 'Nutritional deficiency diseases: A survey of scurvy, rickets and iron-deficiency anemia', in Iscan, M.Y. and Kennedy, K.A.R. (eds.), *Reconstruction of life from the skeleton*, New York, 201–22.

Von den Driesch, A. 1976. 'A Guide to the Measurement of Animal Bones from Archaeological Sites: as developed by the Institut für Palaeoanatomie, Domestikationsforschung und Geschichte der Tiermedizin of the University of Munich', *Peabody Museum Bulletin* 1.

Provisioning and Diet in Hamwic (Mid-Saxon Southampton): New Data and New Perspectives

Ben Jervis

Excavations have taken place in *Hamwic*, mid-Saxon Southampton, since the 1940s (Morton 1992, 9), producing a large dataset including massive quantities of faunal remains and pottery. This paper combines the data from previous analysis of these finds with data from the author's recent analysis of the *Hamwic* pottery, to provide new perspectives on the provisioning and diet of the settlement and its population.

Archaeological background

Hamwic, located on the banks of the River Itchen, to the east of the site of the later medieval town of Southampton, was founded in the seventh century and functioned as a *wic* trading centre, part of an international network of similar settlements around northern Europe (Morton 1992, 26; Cowie and Hill 2001) (Figure 9.1a).

The settlement was planned, with a network of metalled streets and clearly defined tenement plots. Waste management appears to have been well organized, with both ceramic and faunal evidence indicating the presence of middens, which were re-deposited into pits (Jervis 2011, 252–4). However, whilst potentially blurring any spatial patterning, waste does not appear to have moved huge distances, as significant patterning is still evident in the archaeological data. The finds from the settlement provide evidence of craft production, including antler, metal and glass working, as well as evidence of international trade (see Morton 1992; Andrews 1997). Many excavations have taken place within the area of *Hamwic*, which underlies modern St Mary's and Northam, ranging from small evaluations to large open area excavations (see Morton 1992, 5).

Diet in Hamwic

The best evidence for diet comes from the analysis of the large quantities of faunal remains (Bourdillon 1980; Bourdillon 1984; Hamilton-Dyer 2005). Both these and environmental evidence from the *Hamwic* excavations are relatively homogenous across the settlement (Hagen 2005, 356). In all assemblages cattle (accounting for around half the animals present; Bourdillon 1994, 124) and pig dominate the faunal material, with a small quantity of sheep being present. Wild birds and animals are very rare (Bourdillon 1980, 183), for example domestic fowl and geese appear to outnumber wild varieties by a ratio of 1:30 (Bourdillon 1994, 122). Fish, mainly from the local estuaries, was exploited across the settlement and throughout its period of occupation

Provisioning and Diet in Hamwic

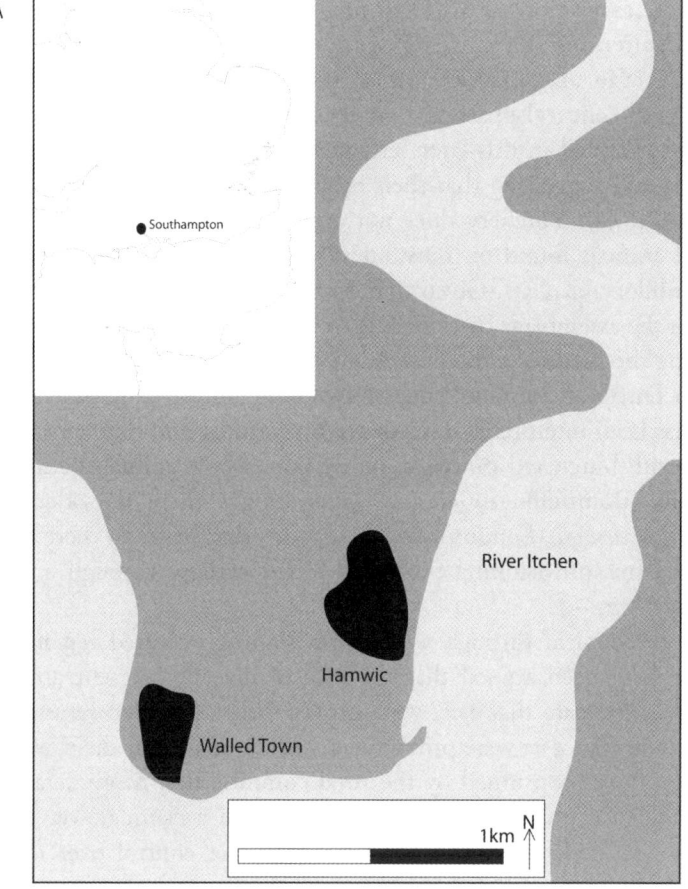

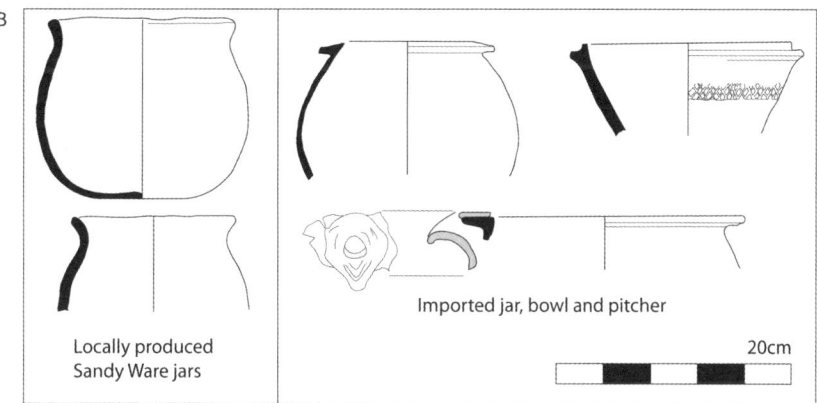

Figure 9.1. b) The location of Hamwic within Southampton; b) Typical ceramic vessels from Hamwic (redrawn from Timby 1988).

(ibid.). The large excavations at Six Dials presented the first opportunity to explore the chronological patterning of faunal remains and a decline in pig numbers in relation to cow, from a ratio of 3.4 cattle:1 pig in the earlier phase to 8.1 cattle:1 pig in the later (ninth–tenth century) phase was noted. Sheep were also less common and older, animals were consumed in this later settlement phase, attesting to the importance of the wool trade and suggesting that their meat was something of a secondary product (Bourdillon 1984, 93). Butchery does not appear to have been specialized, with the same parts of animals found on most sites, having been butchered in a fairly rough fashion (Bourdillon 1984, 45). Given that no body parts are particularly under or over represented in the assemblage, it is likely that animals were brought to *Hamwic* on the hoof, matching the picture at the East Anglian *wic* of Ipswich (Crabtree 1996). This is in contrast to European *wic* sites, such as Dorestad and Hedeby, where an absence of cattle skulls has been interpreted as evidence for farming and butchery in the environs of the ports, with butchered carcasses, rather than whole animals being brought into the settlements (Bourdillon 1994, 122). Interestingly, there is evidence of neonate animals from *Lundenwic* (London), which suggests that here too there may have been some satellite farms provisioning the *wic* directly, perhaps through a market system (Hamerow 2007, 222–3).

The exact mechanism through which provisioning occurred remains a matter of debate. It has long been argued that the lack of diversity present and the presence of older animals indicate that *wics* were provisioned from food rents levied to rural communities, and that *wics* were provisioned with animals past their useful life, whilst more prime meat was consumed by the rural communities. More detailed reading of the zooarchaeological evidence does not support such a claim however (Sykes 2006, 63–4), with towns perhaps having a greater degree of control over their provisions than previously thought, although with the poorly developed market system limiting the choice available. This is not a debate which the new ceramic data presented here can greatly contribute, however it does allow us to explore some of the complexities of provisioning systems more generally, particularly within *Hamwic*.

Food crops also appear to have been imported into towns; however the presence of quern stones demonstrates that grains were processed within *Hamwic*. Wheat consumption appears to have increased in the later phases, although the absolute quantities of other grains did not decrease (Biddle unpub.). Amongst remains from more recent excavations at St Mary's Stadium the remains of cabbage were identified (Hunter 2005).

In two of the excavated cemeteries, at Marine Parade (SOU 13) and Clifford Street (SOU 31), there is a high incidence of caries, suggestive of a diet rich in carbohydrates (Pay unpublished). At Clifford Street (SOU 31), the high levels of strontium in the teeth suggest that the diet was relatively meat free and high sodium levels suggest that fish were an important part of the diet. Males appear to have a higher incidence of calculus on the teeth, suggestive of a more protein rich diet than the females. Perhaps males had better access to meat than females. Further evidence is provided by the cemetery at St Mary's Stadium (SOU 1019). Here, in an early cemetery, there is a very low incidence of caries, suggesting a meat-rich diet (McKinley 2005), perhaps related to the fact that *Hamwic* appears to have developed from a high status royal 'vill', based on the presence of furnished burials and historical references (Hinton 2005, 75–7). The evidence from the human remains can tentatively be used to suggest that food consumption reflected, or played an active role in the construction of, social groups within the town, perhaps along lines of class or gender in the early phase of the settlement at least. This contrasts the relative homogeneity in the faunal assemblage however. This may in part be due to depositional practices, which have blurred distinctions in material culture patterning, although the ceramic evidence (discussed below) suggests that the effect of this is limited. Rather, it should be considered that the skeletal remains relate to an early phase of the settlement when social distinction may have been more marked, as elites emphasized their authority through the foundation of this settlement. Furthermore, skeletal material offers a higher degree of resolution, allowing us to see what individuals were consuming, whilst, at best, faunal remains can only provide this data at a household level failing to account for differential consumption within a domestic unit.

Studies of the Hamwic pottery

There have been two major studies of the *Hamwic* pottery. The first, undertaken by Hodges (1981), focussed on defining the imported wares and tracking the trade routes in which *Hamwic* participated. The second study, undertaken by Timby (1988), concentrated more on defining the locally produced wares in terms of source and chronology. These studies have led to the definition of 8 groups of locally produced wares, which can broadly be split into three ceramic phases (Table 9.1). These are typically present as jars, with everted rims and sagging bases, often termed cooking pots; however in reality they had a multitude of functions (Figure 9.1b). Imported wares have been identified as principally coming from northern France, Flanders and the

Table 9.1. Hamwic ceramic phases.

Phase	Date Range	Typical Pottery
1	*c.* 7th–8th	Organic/chaff tempered wares.
2	*c.* 8th–9th	sandy wares, chalk-tempered wares.
3	*c.* 9th–10th	Mixed grit tempered wares, flint tempered wares, shelly wares.
	Wares of uncertain date	Most imports, calcite tempered and igneous rock tempered wares.

Rhineland, however there are a small number of sherds from further afield, including the Alsace. These are present in a wider range of forms including jars, pitchers and bowls (Figure 9.1b). My study has reinterpreted this data to better understand the distribution

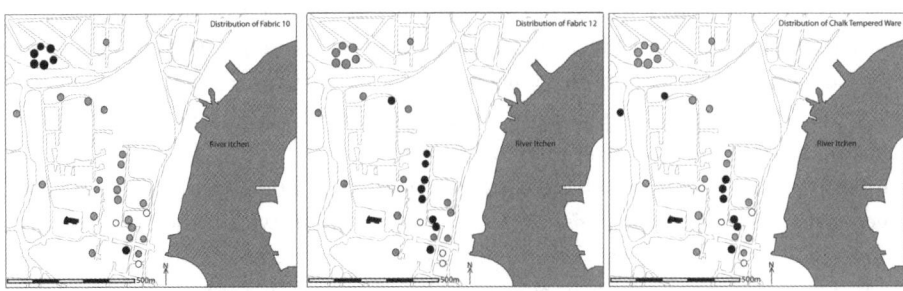

Figure 9.2: Distribution of phase 2 wares within Hamwic. Black dots denote fabric over-represented. Grey dots denote ware present. Dot size denotes size of site assemblage (see table 9.3 for data).

mechanisms behind these wares within the settlement and I have also re-examined some of the pottery in order to undertake usewear analysis (see also Jervis 2011a).

Methodology

The study of use alteration patterns is rarely undertaken on medieval pottery, however this study demonstrates that if undertaken systematically it has the potential to provide useful results. The methodology adopted follows that devised by Skibo (1992), whilst also taking into account the findings of Moorhouse's (1983) study of usewear on medieval pottery from Sandal Castle (Yorkshire). Sherds were selected from the most secure contexts, where pottery was least fragmented and were studied under a x10 binocular microscope. Two strands of use data were recorded, the first were attrition indicators, including indicators of physical processes such as abrasion and scratching and indicators of chemical attrition, such as pitting resulting from a reaction between the contents and the vessel wall (for example, through processes such as brewing; see Perry 2011), which provide evidence of stirring, movement and the use of lids or pot boilers. The second strand were sooting patterns, providing evidence of cooking methods. During analysis a high number of combinations of various indicators were identified, however each group generally consisted of very small numbers of sherds, or, in many cases, single sherds. Therefore a more simple approach has been adopted, with vessels being categorized as follows:

Cooking vessels demonstrate evidence of sooting and/or spalling, suggestive of use over a fire.

Preparation vessels do not demonstrate evidence of use over a fire, but have internal attrition.

Storage/serving vessels exhibit no evidence of use, or only exterior attrition. A differentiation between storage and serving vessels can be made based upon a vessel's fabric and form.

Because the assemblages are generally quite fragmented, some sherds may not exhibit signs of use, meaning that storage/serving vessels are likely to be over-represented and cooking/preparation vessels under-represented. It can be assumed, based on the fact that the level of fragmentation is fairly similar across the settlement (Jervis 2011b, 221), that this effect is consistent. Therefore, whilst perhaps not offering a wholly accurate reconstruction of ceramic use, the analysis has created an index of use, which can be used to compare use patterns through space and time. Further to this analysis, a sample of 24 sherds were submitted for residue analysis using standard GC–MS techniques (see Barclay 2001).

Results
Provisioning

By studying the distribution of local pottery we can examine how resources were exchanged within the settlement. The best evidence comes from the second ceramic phase, probably dating to the eighth–ninth centuries (Table 9.1), when the settlement was at its peak. The most abundant pottery in this phase are sandy wares, which were locally produced (Timby 1988, 112; table 2). In general terms, the two main fabrics (10 and 12) can be demonstrated to have concentrated distributions in particular areas of the settlement, suggesting that these products were redistributed at a relatively localized level. Table 9.2 shows the composition of assemblages at each site in *Hamwic*. In the north, around Six Dials in particular, fabric 10 accounts for relatively high proportions of assemblages in relation to fabric 12. In contrast, fabric 12 is more abundant at sites around Melbourne Street and Chapel Road, towards the south of the settlement. Table 9.3 shows the spread (the proportion of the total of each fabric present at each site) of these wares across *Hamwic*.

By comparing these figures with the size of an assemblage, and thus the proportion of the *Hamwic* total present, it is possible to see if wares appear over- or under-represented at a site, working on the assumption that if no patterning was present there would be a strong correlation between the percentage of a given fabric present and the percentage of the entire assemblage present within a particular phase, at a particular site. A similar pattern is apparent in this analysis. For example at SOU 31 (Six Dials) 23% of the total fabric 10 is present, at a site which accounts for only 16% of the phase 2 assemblage. Similarly at SOU 4 (Melbourne Street) 9% of the total fabric 12 is present, at a site which accounts for only 3% of the phase 2 assemblage (see Figures 9.2a and 9.2b). Chalk-tempered wares are also present in this phase. These were produced outside of the settlement, probably in the Winchester area (Timby 1988, 82) and are found settlement wide. Generally, the proportion of the total chalk-tempered wares present at a site reflects the proportion of the total phase 2 assemblage at that site (Table 9.3; Figure 9.2c), therefore they are relatively evenly spread through *Hamwic*. This spatial patterning suggests that despite patterns of re-deposition, it is still possible to identify genuine patterning in the material culture and food remains present in *Hamwic*. It is

Table 9.2. *The composition of phase 2 pottery assemblages at sites in Hamwic (by weight in grammes).*

Area	SOU	Sandy Fabric 10	Fabric 12	Other sandy wares	Chalk-tempered wares	Early mixed grit tempered	Total (g)
Centre	43	37%	27%	35%	1%		116
Clifford Street	15	12%	16%	21%	35%	17%	7016
	32	12%	13%	22%	35%	18%	7709
	39	18%	5%	10%	47%	20%	3143
Marine Parade	10		100%				8
	13	13%	25%	31%	18%	13%	248
Melbourne St.	1	19%	22%	32%	26%	1%	5617
	4	16%	50%	25%	8%	1%	5841
	5	9%	22%	14%	44%	11%	4235
	6	16%	41%	5%	33%	6%	2114
	20	2%	29%	46%	13%	10%	3680
N. of Chapel Rd.	7	14%	42%	27%	11%	6%	557
	8	3%	17%	59%	11%	10%	1231
	11	21%	14%	14%	27%	23%	4982
	18	7%	37%	3%	53%		630
	33	8%	8%	23%	46%	15%	15671
	40	100%					29
Northumberland Rd.	19	28%	4%	22%	44%	2%	330
Six Dials	23	30%	12%	34%	22%	2%	2513
	24	48%	11%	15%	22%	4%	25106
	26	41%	1%	18%	29%	10%	15368
	30	25%	7%	37%	26%	5%	16891
	31	41%	11%	19%	23%	6%	33470
	169	36%	14%	19%	20%	10%	21989
S. Periphery	14	28%	38%	13%	16%	5%	14033
	16	13%		80%	7%		99
	17	<1%	9%	16%	68%	6%	6427
	22			33%		67%	12
W. Periphery	36	17%	12%	14%	42%	14%	7181
	99	23%	11%	31%	29%	6%	5990
Total		28%	15%	21%	28%	9%	212236

Table 9.3. The spread of phase 2 wares through Hamwic (weight in grammes); see explanation of method in text.

Area	SOU	Chalk-tempered ware	Sandy wares		All phase 2 wares
			10	12	
Centre	43	<1%	<1%	<1%	<1%
Clifford Street	15	4%	1%	4%	3%
	32	5%	2%	3%	4%
	39	3%	1%	<1%	1%
Marine Parade	10			<1%	<1%
	13	<1%	<1%	<1%	<1%
Melbourne Street	1	2%	2%	4%	3%
	4	1%	2%	9%	3%
	5	3%	1%	3%	2%
	6	1%	1%	3%	1%
	20	1%	<1%	4%	2%
N. of Chapel Rd.	7	<1%	<1%	1%	<1%
	8	<1%	<1%	1%	1%
	11	2%	2%	2%	2%
	18	1%	<1%	1%	<1%
	33	12%	2%	4%	7%
	40		<1%		<1%
Northumberland Road	19	<1%	<1%	<1%	<1%
Six Dials	23	1%	1%	1%	1%
	24	9%	20%	9%	12%
	26	8%	11%	1%	7%
	30	7%	7%	4%	8%
	31	13%	23%	12%	16%
	169	7%	13%	10%	10%
Southern Periphery	14	4%	7%	17%	7%
	16	<1%	<1%		<1%
	17	7%	<1%	2%	3%
	22				<1%
Western Periphery	36	5%	2%	3%	3%
	99	3%	2%	2%	3%
Total (g)		59303	59008	30843	212236

possible that these entered the settlement as containers (see below). Their distribution would seem to illustrate the presence of a second redistribution mechanism, whereby some resources were marketed or exchanged at a settlement-wide scale. The relatively clear definition in distribution of the local products suggests that the homogenous spatial patterning in the faunal remains is genuine, and not the result of redeposition. We can use this information to infer that resources brought from outside had a different pattern of redistribution to those produced within or close to it. Certain imported wares have very localized distributions, suggesting that they were products brought to *Hamwic* not for trade, but for use by immigrant merchants or their households. It is possible that some exotic foodstuffs entered *Hamwic* by these means too, but this cannot be demonstrated with any certainty.

Cooking methods and pottery use
In tempered 1, that is the seventh and early eighth centuries, we can observe a general consistency in the cooking methods used, however it must be stressed the number of sherds examined is very small. Cooking vessels typically display dull black/grey sooty deposits, which form when a vessel is placed close to the heat (Skibo 2013, 90–2), all over their bodies, which is demonstrative of placement in or close to a fire during cooking. There are some areas of difference however. In the north of the settlement (SOU 24), glossy black sooting, formed when the vessel wall is cooler (Skibo 2013, 90–2), is more common (Table 9.4; Figure 9.3a).

Table 9.4. Pottery use in phase 1 (maximum number of vessels).

SOU	4	11	14	24	169
Cooking (Black Carbonized)	14	6	9	4	2
Cooking (Glossy Black)	8	0	7	4	1
Cooking (Spalling only)	2	0	0	0	0
Storage	31	12	23	8	7
Preparation	21	9	21	4	7
Total (Max. Vessels)	76	27	60	20	17

It appears therefore that there may be variation in cooking practices in different areas of the settlement, perhaps the result of *Hamwic*'s community being formed of people from a variety of settlements, who had learnt to cook in different ways (see Jervis 2011a, 247). This conclusion, that the same foodstuffs were cooked in different ways, could not be reached without integrated analysis, demonstrating the value of such an approach in the study of diet and cuisine. The distribution of storage vessels in this phase suggests that every household had a surplus of some kind to store, perhaps relating to the wider exchange network. Vessels demonstrating evidence of use in food preparation or processing appear focussed at the periphery (SOUs 11, 14, 169). This may be related to people in these areas participating in more agricultural activity. Alternatively, a different cooking method may have been used in this area, such as the use of pot boilers, which is attested to in contemporary sources (Hagen 2005, 287).

Table 9.5. Sandy ware use (phase 2) (maximum number of vessels).

SOU	1	4	5	6	11	14	24	26	30	31	169	1019
Cooking (Black Carbonised)	12	35	25	17	24	178	15	151	11	63	21	20
Cooking (Glossy Black)	6	12	11	6	5	67	24	36	10	36	22	3
Cooking (Spalling Only)	2	2	1	1	1	0	5	2	0	5	1	0
Storage	33	61	44	37	57	369	74	285	25	261	55	23
Preparation	18	32	24	25	38	129	39	95	24	93	52	9
Total (Max. Vessels)	71	142	105	86	125	743	157	569	70	458	151	55

Table 9.6. Chalk-tempered ware use (phase 2) (maximum number of vessels).

SOU	1	4	5	6	11	14	24	26	30	31	169	1019
Cooking (Black Carbonised)	2	3	13	1	9	29	12	8	2	16	15	6
Cooking (Glossy Black)	7	2	10	0	10	9	13	10	1	12	22	4
Cooking (Spalling Only)	2	0	2	0	5	0	0	2	0	5	13	0
Storage	33	10	63	8	68	124	48	51	12	113	46	8
Preparation	7	1	25	4	33	39	41	30	4	45	33	4
Total (Max. Vessels)	51	16	113	13	125	201	114	101	19	191	129	22

In the second phase there is increased uniformity in ceramic use across the settlement. Sandy wares seem to have had a range of functions, but were particularly popular as cooking and preparation vessels (Table 9.5; Figure 9.3b). Duller black sooty deposits are the most common evidence of cooking, but glossy black sooting being more widespread than in phase 1, however there remains a distinction between the north-west and south-east of the settlement, perhaps reflecting the inheritance of cooking techniques through domestic scale learning patterns (Jervis 2011, 249). The greater homogeneity in the use profiles of assemblages throughout the settlement suggests a cohesive community organized around a relatively egalitarian provisioning system, reflecting the faunal

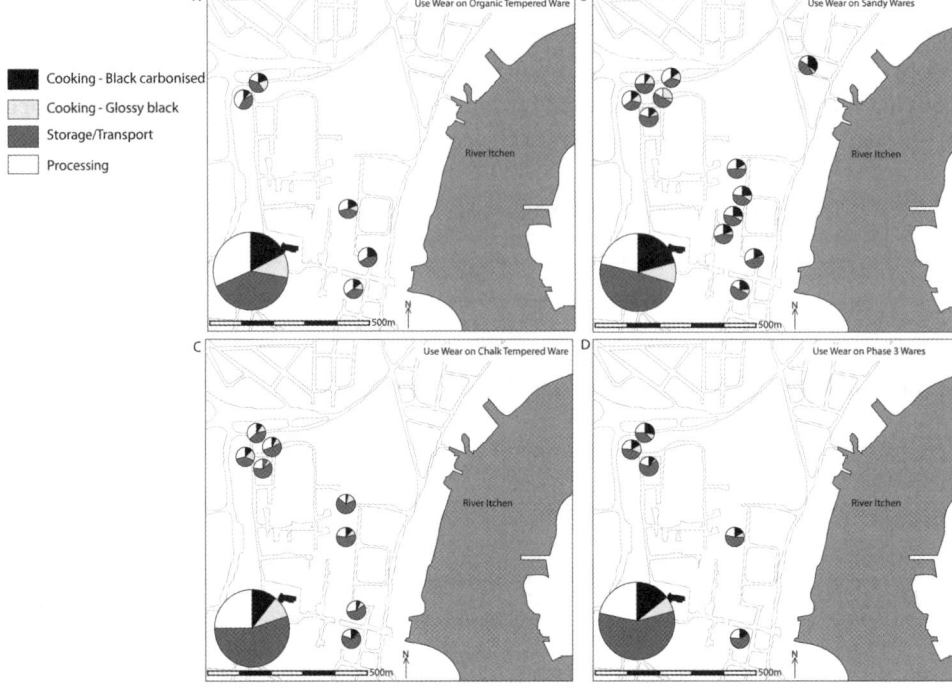

Figure 9.3. Ceramic use patterns in Hamwic: a) Organic tempered wares (phase 1); b) sandy wares (phase 2); c) chalk-tempered wares (phase 2); d) phase 3 wares (see tables 4–7 for data).

Table 9.7. Phase 3 vessel use (maximum number of vessels).

SOU	1	4	5	6	11	14	24	26	30	31	169	1019
Cooking (Black Carbonised)	1	4	43	0	20	54	40	17	4	93	63	13
Cooking (Glossy Black)	0	2	15	2	5	9	14	9	0	33	56	7
Cooking (Spalling Only)	1	3	3	2	4	3	4	2	0	17	9	1
Storage	6	12	262	1	32	209	54	68	8	563	167	10
Preparation	2	5	70	4	18	83	36	25	11	170	88	8
Total (Max. Vessels)	10	26	393	9	79	358	148	121	23	876	383	39

evidence. The chalk-tempered wares occupy a more uncertain functional position. The high proportion used for storage suggests that they may have originally been used as containers. There is a higher degree of variability in the quantity of these vessels used as cooking or preparation vessels, and this may relate to the availability of local wares, or the use of these vessels for whatever function was required as they became available (Table 9.6; Figure 9.3c).

The final ceramic phase (phase 3), is characterized by the use of gritty wares (Table 9.1). In this phase use patterns appear more localized. Across the settlement a similar method of cooking seems to have been favoured, leading to the creation of black/grey carbonized deposits (Table 9.7; Figure 9.3d).

As before, glossy black deposits are rarer (Figure 9.4). There is no consistency in the sizes or forms of vessels used for cooking. Varying proportions of vessels were used in preparation and storage. The range of use profiles present when compared to ceramic phase 2 indicates provisioning may not have been so egalitarian and that people may have had different needs to be met by ceramic vessels. The high proportion of storage vessels indicates that there were still surpluses to store, but the continued presence of preparation vessels throughout the settlement may indicate that these were processed at a household level. This period relates to the reorganization of *Hamwic* (Hall 2000, 127), possibly a time of economic stress, perhaps reflected in the decrease in pig (a purely meat-bearing animal) and sheep (perhaps as elites sought to exercise greater control over wool supply) consumption in the settlement, with this context perhaps being conducive to increased storage of surpluses and the distribution and consumption of these within smaller social groups.

Finally, we can consider the role of imported wares in food consumption. For the purposes of this paper these have been grouped into 4 categories. Greywares, Blackwares and Whitewares are common throughout the settlement. The fourth group contains less common types, found at only a few sites. Based on their distribution, greywares appear to have been exchanged on the open market, and this may explain why they are present as cooking pots at nearly every site considered (Table 9.8). Blackwares were less commonly used as cooking vessels. Where they were, it is at sites with high quantities of other imported cooking pots (Table 9.8). There are particularly high quantities of imported cooking vessels at Melbourne Street (SOU 4 and SOU 5) and, to a lesser degree, at Six Dials (SOU 24 and SOU 26). These are sites with a particularly wide range of imports, which suggests that they were involved in the more personal exchange mechanisms, perhaps including the homes of immigrants or local people with continental ties. At Melbourne Street there are a particularly low number of phase 3 cooking vessels, perhaps suggesting that this was the home of an immigrant during this phase (Table 9.8), who engaged in Continental, rather than local cooking practices. Elsewhere, local cooking vessels appear to have been used alongside imported ones, or the archaeological record is too coarse to differentiate between household units, partly due to the probability that middens functioned as repository for a neighbourhood, rather than a single household's waste, with material from one house being distributed into negative features associated with different households. The attrition on imported wares demonstrates that these were used for a range of functions. They generally exhibit no or only exterior attrition (perhaps resulting from transit), suggesting a function as storage vessels, although some, such as spouted pitchers, may have been serving vessels. This could have been their principle function, as this role was not catered for by the local wares (Brown 1997, 110–11). The presence of serving vessels across *Hamwic* (and their rarity outside of the settlement) demonstrates that people in *Hamwic* engaged in particularly cosmopolitan practices. Whilst many households partook in public consumption practices, the use of imported cooking vessels in some households may have served to maintain a different identity, perhaps of ethnicity.

Table 9.8. Imported vessel use (maximum number of vessels).

	SOU	1	4	5	6	11	14	24	26	30	31	169	1019
Blackware	Cooking (Black Carbonised)					3	1					1	
	Cooking (Glossy Black)		2	2		1	1						
	Cooking (Spalling Only)												
	Storage/Serving	1	2	1	13		7		5	1	7	2	2
	Preparation			4	10	4	21	5	5	5	7	6	2
	Total (Max. Vessels)	1	4	7	23	8	30	5	10	6	14	9	4
Greyware	Cooking (Black Carbonised)		2	2		4	6	2	3		5	6	
	Cooking (Glossy Black)			1	2		2	1	1			1	1
	Cooking (Spalling Only)			1			1		2		1	2	
	Storage/Serving		1	3	3	5	21	11	9	1	21	6	11
	Preparation		4	9	5	17	17	9	19		13	16	5
	Total (Max. Vessels)		7	16	10	26	47	23	34	1	40	31	17
Whiteware	Cooking (Black Carbonised)						4						1
	Cooking (Glossy Black)						2						
	Cooking (Spalling Only)						1						
	Storage/Serving						7				2	2	1
	Preparation					2	8						
	Total (Max. Vessels)					2	22				2	2	2

Provisioning and Diet in Hamwic

Other Import	Cooking (Black Carbonised)	1	2	2	1	1	4	3	7	2	6	2	
	Cooking (Glossy Black)		2	3	1	1	1	1	2		1	2	
	Cooking (Spalling Only)		2	3					2	1	3	3	
	Storage/Serving	1	4	6	7	7	12	2	6	6	18	17	5
	Preparation	1		3	2	3	7	4	8	6	15	6	1
	Total (Max. Vessels)	3	10	17	11	12	24	10	25	15	43	30	6
Total	Cooking (Black Carbonised)	1	4	4	1	8	15	5	10	2	11	9	1
	Cooking (Glossy Black)		4	6	3	2	6	2	3		1	3	1
	Cooking (Spalling Only)		2	4			2		4	1	4	5	
	Storage/Serving	2	7	10	23	12	47	13	20	8	48	27	19
	Preparation	1	4	16	17	26	53	18	32	11	35	28	8
	Total (Max. Vessels)	4	21	40	44	48	123	38	69	22	99	72	29

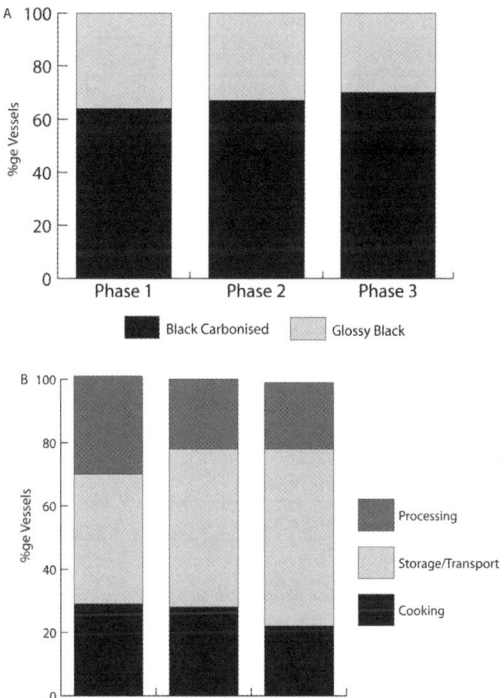

Figure 9.4: A) Temporal trends in sooting type in Hamwic. B) Temporal trends in the pottery function in Hamwic (see tables 4–7 for data).

Table 9.9: Results of residue analysis (after Baeten et al. in press).

Sample	Fabric	Site	Fish	Animal Fat	Vegetable Foodstuffs	Beeswax
1	10 (sandy ware)	24	-	-	-	-
2	10	31	-	Ruminant	Cabbage	-
3	11 (Organic-tempered sandy ware)	24	-	-	-	-
4	11	1	-	Ruminant	Present	-
5	12 (sandy ware)	1	-	Ruminant	Present	-
6	12	4	-	Present	Present	-
7	11	11	?	Ruminant	Present	-
8	59 (Gritty ware)	8	-	Ruminant	Cabbage	-
9	40 (chalk-tempered ware)	24	Present	Ruminant	Present	-
10	12	4	-	-	-	-
11	10	14	Present	Ruminant	Cabbage	-
12	10	4	Present	-	Cabbage	-
13	10	14	?	Present	Cabbage	-
14	10	4	-	Ruminant	Present	-
15	12	14	-	Ruminant	Present	-
16	10	14	-	-	Cabbage	-
17	12	14	-	Ruminant	Cabbage	-
18	40	4	-	Ruminant	-	Present
19	12	4	-	Ruminant	Present	-
20	40	31	-	-	-	-
21	sandy ware	31	-	-	-	-
22	sandy ware	31	-	-	-	-
23	sandy ware	31	-	Ruminant	Cabbage	-
24	sandy ware	31	-	Ruminant	Cabbage	-

New insights into food consumption[1]

GC–MS analysis of a sample of 24 sherds was undertaken (Baeten et al. in press). The majority of the sherds examined demonstrated evidence of ruminant fat and fish indicators and correspond therefore with the faunal and archaeobotanical evidence from excavations (Table 9.9). Importantly a number of sherds display evidence of food mixing. This evidence includes the mixing of vegetable and meat foodstuffs in the creation of stews, a process which can only be implied rather than directly inferred through the study of environmental remains alone. Interestingly, leafy vegetables are considered not to have been a major component of Anglo-Saxon diet by Blinkhorn (2012, 51), based on the results of GC–MS analysis of contemporary Ipswich ware. Therefore, the results of the *Hamwic* analysis perhaps point to regional consumption patterns, in which leafy vegetables may be an indicator of a distinctively Wessex diet, which may prove a fruitful line for future research. Such regionality may also be seen in the differences in the age of death of the animals consumed in *Lundenwic* (see above). Whilst the lipid biomarkers provide the evidence for food mixing, the sooting patterns, indicating the placement of pots into the embers, provides evidence for the cooking method (see also Baetens et al. in press). Marine and ruminant fats were also found together in two vessels. Whilst this may relate to vessel re-use, it is possible that the lipid analysis has provided evidence of the cooking of fish in milk or butter, a technique recorded in contemporary texts (Hagen 2006, 294). Finally, the interpretation of chalk-tempered wares as storage or transport vessels is supported by the identification of beeswax in one of these vessels. This may indicate the sealing of a porous vessel to make it suitable for the long term storage of liquids, or alternatively may indicate the presence of honey, an important sweetener and preservative in the period, which was common in food rents and has been found in a significant quantity of Ipswich ware vessels (Blinkhorn 2012, 49).

Conclusions

Previous analysis of the faunal, environmental and human remains from *Hamwic* provided a rough picture of diet in the settlement. It had been suggested that diet was relatively homogenous, although the human remains did suggest there may have been some differentiation along class or gender lines. Pottery analysis has added further evidence to the discussion. The study of pottery distribution has demonstrated that several exchange mechanisms were present within the settlement, operating at different scales. Furthermore, analysis of the distribution of chalk-tempered ware inside the settlement, and the analysis of absorbed organic residue, indicates that these vessels entered *Hamwic* as containers, the contents of which appear to have been widely used. Analysis of cooking practices has demonstrated that in phase 2, when the settlement was at its peak, people cooked in similar ways, whilst households appear to have had similar proportions of cooking, storage and preparation vessels. In phase 1 cooking practices appear generally similar, although there is the suggestion in the north that cooking vessels may have been kept cooler, whilst in the south pot boilers may have been used. Alternatively, it is possible that the south of the settlement was semi-rural in nature and people here had a distinct economic role in the processing of foodstuffs.

In phase 3 there is similarity in the cooking practices used, but the increase in the number of storage vessels and the seemingly localized pattern of processing, when coupled with the changes in the faunal assemblage, can perhaps be seen as indicative of a time of stress within the settlement, perhaps as centralized redistribution broke down and sheep and pig became scarce, it became necessary for provisioning to be organized at a household, rather than settlement wide, level. The imported wares illustrate a further level of social distinction. Most households appear to have utilized imported serving vessels, and this served to mark the population of *Hamwic* as distinctly cosmopolitan in comparison with rural settlements in southern England. The use of specific imported cooking pots appears more localized however, and this may be indicative of certain immigrant members of the population maintaining their distinct identity through foreign cooking practices. Some idiosyncrasies in the sooting on local wares may also be indicative of immigrants attempting to apply foreign cooking methods to local pottery. Finally, the preliminary GC–MS results provide exciting evidence that whilst the core elements of diet may have been relatively homogenous, particular households may have used certain flavouring agents in their foods, possibly indicating differences in taste, perhaps related to the socio-economic context of each home.

Acknowledgements

The GC–MS analysis was funded by the Society for Medieval Archaeology (Eric Fletcher Fund) and The University of Southampton, and was undertaken by Dr Jan Baeten at KU Leuven. This research is part of an AHRC funded doctoral project. I would like to thank Duncan Brown, Matthew Garner, Dr. James Morris, Dr Katherine Robbins my supervisor, Dr. Andrew Jones and the anonymous reviewer, for their assistance and support at various stages of this research. I would also like to thank Karen Wardley, Sian Iles and Gill Woolrich for providing access to the *Hamwic* collections.

Note

1. This paper was completed prior to the publication of the results of the Ipswich ware project (Blinkhorn 2012). Whilst the results are mentioned in this section, it is intended that a more comprehensive comparison of the results of analysis of Ipswich ware and material from Hamwic will form the basis of a future publication.

References

Andrews, P. 1997. *Excavations at* Hamwic *Volume 2: Six Dials*, CBA Research Report 109.

Baeten, J., Jervis, B., De Vos, D. and Waelkens, M. In press. 'Molecular Evidence for the Mixing of Meat, Fish and Vegetables in Anglo-Saxon Coarseware from Hamwic, UK', *Archaeometry*.

Barclay, K. 2001. *Scientific Analysis of Archaeological Ceramics*, Oxford.

Biddle, B. Unpublished. *A Comparison of the Plant Remains from Archaeological Excavations in Southampton, with a Special Reference to the Seeds*, Unpublished report in Southampton City Museum.

Blinkhorn, P. 2012. *The Ipswich Ware Project: Ceramics, Trade and Society in Middle Saxon England*, Medieval Pottery Research Group Occasional Paper 7.

Bourdillon, J. 1980. 'Town Life and Animal Husbandry in the Southampton Area, as Suggested by the Excavated Bones', *Proceedings of the Hampshire Field Club Archaeological Society* 36, 181–191.

Bourdillon, J. 1984. *Animal Bone from Saxon Southampton: The Six Dials Variability Survey*. Report to the Ancient Monuments Laboratory.

Brown, D. 1997. 'The Social Significance of Imported Medieval Pottery', in Blinkhorn, P. and Cumberpatch, C. (eds.), *Not so Much a Pot: More a Way of Life*, Oxford, 95–112.

Cowie, R and Hill, D (eds.). 2001. *Wics: The early medieval trading centres of northern Europe*, Sheffield.

Crabtree, P. 1996. 'Production and consumption in an early complex society: animal use in Middle Saxon East Anglia', *World Archaeology* 28, 58–75.

Hagen, A. 2005. *Anglo-Saxon Food and Drink. Production, Processing, Distribution and Consumption*, Hockwold cum Wilton.

Hall, R. 2000. 'The Decline of the *Wic*?', in Slater, T. (ed.), *Towns in Decline AD 100–1600*, Aldershot.

Hamerow, H. 2007. 'Agrarian production and the emporia of mid Saxon England, ca AD 650–850', in Henning, J. (ed.), *Post-Roman Towns and Settlement in Europe and Byzantium. Vol. 1 The Heirs of the Roman West*, Berlin, 219–32.

Hamilton-Dyer, S. 2005. 'Animal bones', in Birbeck, V. (ed.), *The Origins of Mid-Saxon Southampton. Excavations at the Friends Provident St Mary's Stadium 1998–2000*, Salisbury, 140–53.

Hinton, D.A. 2005. *Gold and Gilt, Pots and Pins*, Oxford.

Hodges, R. 1981. *The Hamwih Pottery: The local and imported wares from 30 year's excavations at Middle Saxon Southampton and their European context*, CBA Research Report 37.

Hunter, K. 2005. 'Charred Plant Remains', in Birbeck, V. (ed.), *The Origins of Mid-Saxon Southampton. Excavations at the Friends Provident St Mary's Stadium 1998–2000*, Salisbury, 163–73.

Jervis, B. 2011a. 'A Patchwork of People, Pots and Places: Material Engagements and the Construction of 'the social' in Hamwic (Anglo-Saxon Southampton), UK', *Journal of Social Archaeology* 11(3), 239–65.

Jervis, B. 2011b. *Placing Pottery: An Actor-led Approach to the Use and Perception of Medieval Pottery in Southampton and its Region cAD700–1400*, PhD Diss. University of Southampton.

McKinley, J. 2005. 'Skeletal human remains', in Birbeck, V. (ed.), *The Origins of Mid-Saxon Southampton. Excavations at the Friends Provident St Mary's Stadium 1998–2000*, Salisbury, 47–52.

Morton, A. 1982. *Excavations at* Hamwic *Volume 1: Excavations 1946–83, excluding Six Dials and Melbourne Street*, CBA Research Report 84.

Pay, S. Unpublished. *The Indicators of Diet and Health from the Human Bones Recovered from* Hamwic *(SOUs 13 and 31)*, Unpublished report in Southampton City Museum.

Perry, G. 2011. 'Beer, Butter and Burial. The Pre-Burial Origins of Cremation Urns from the Early Anglo-Saxon Cemetery of Cleatham, North Lincolnshire', *Medieval Ceramics* 32, 9–22.

Skibo, J. 1992. *Pottery Function: A use alteration perspective*, New York.

Skibo, J. 2013. *Understanding Pottery Function*, New York.

Sykes, N. 2006. 'From *Cu* and *Sceap* to *Beffe* and *Motton*', in Woolgar, C., Serjeantson, D. and Waldron, T. (eds.), *Food in Medieval England. Diet and Nutrition*, Oxford, 56–71.

Timby, J. 1988. 'The Pottery', in Andrews, P (ed.), *The Pottery and Coins from* Hamwic, Southampton City Museums.

Provisioning Shakespeare's Audiences: Food and Drink in the London Playhouses of the Sixteenth and Seventeenth Centuries

Julian M.C. Bowsher
Museum of London Archaeology

The 'Shakespearean period' in the history of English drama stretches between 1567 – when the first identifiable purpose-built playhouse, the Red Lion in Stepney was built by John Brayne, and 1642 – when all theatres, playhouses and other forms of public entertainment were closed down by Parliament as civil war loomed. The physical manifestations of this period were the unique, mostly polygonal, playhouses in London. The playhouses were mostly located in the suburbs, but this is more likely to reflect cheaper rents and wider space rather than Puritan opposition to performance within the City itself. In fact plays were also put on at certain City inns and other indoor venues, ranging from the royal court and the halls of the livery companies and the great magnates of Tudor Britain.

Victualling, particularly drinking, has always played an important part in (early) modern theatre economy. The very location of these theatrical venues, mostly outside the City, lay within areas already home to taverns, brothels, bear-baiting arenas and other forms of dubious entertainment. Rowdy behaviour at the playhouses brought down the heavy hand of the law with frequent demands for their closure and even demolition. Opponents, such as Philip Stubbes in 1583, were quick to associate 'theatres and unclean assemblies' with 'idleness, unthriftiness, whoredom, wantoness, drunkenesss, and what not' (Wickham et al. 2000, 166). Church opposition was particularly acute; in a sermon of October 1623 Thomas Adams railed against the 'Men and women, whose whole employment is, to go from their beds to the tap-house, then to the playhouse, where they make a match for the brothel-house, and from thence to bed again' (Angus 1862, 182).

The buildings
The history of these buildings, and their internal function, has long been an academic subject in its own right but it was only with the arrival of archaeology on the Shakespearean stage that concrete evidence for the shape, size and development of the playhouses, let alone artefactual and ecofactual remains within, emerged. The archaeological aspect of this paper is centred on the outdoor playhouses of which MOLA (Museum of London Archaeology) has investigated the sites of no less than six of them as well as two of the Bankside animal baiting rings – architecturally and,

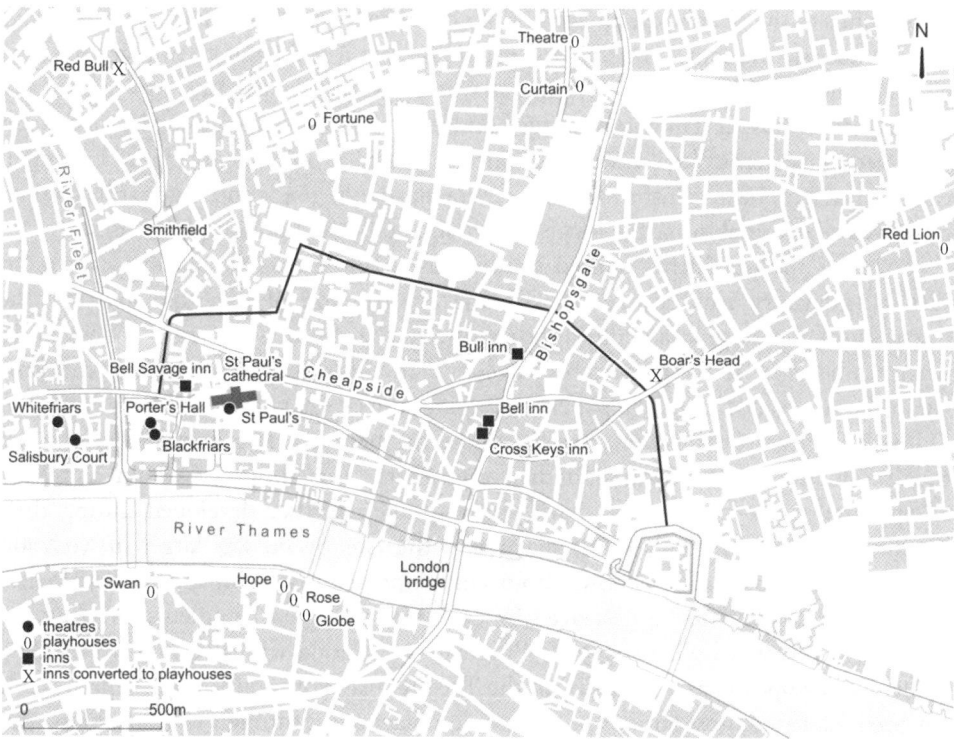

Figure 10.1. Map showing the location of the sites mentiond in the text (Copyright Museum of London Archaeology).

socially similar (for a detailed examination of these buildings and their archaeology, see Bowsher 2012) (Figure 10.1). The archaeological content of this paper is limited to these outdoor playhouses rather than the indoor venues which do not survive. The sites of the City inns have been continuously redeveloped and, where investigated, no associated remains have been unearthed. The indoor theatres, such as the famous Blackfriars, were all (with the possible exception of the Cockpit / Phoenix in Drury Lane) installed within existing buildings and, moreover, on the first floor – leaving little or no archaeological potential.

The exact location of the Red Lion of 1567 is not certain and only a few details of its construction are known, but it does not appear to have functioned as a playhouse for long (Ingram 1992, 102–113). Another early, albeit unnamed, playhouse was located at the small village of Newington Butts in about 1575 under the management (and possibly builder) of an actor Jerome Savage. There are a few details about its life and its location, almost certainly under the roundabout at the Elephant and Castle, but not of its construction. The first proper 'theatrical area' in London was Shoreditch where the Theatre of 1576 and the Curtain of 1577 were located, and small areas of both have been excavated in 2008–11 (Knight 2009) and 2011 respectively. The Theatre, built in the grounds of the dissolved Holywell Priory by Brayne's brother in law James Burbage, was erroneously thought to be the 'first playhouse' but it still retains a primacy in terms of being the first identifiable polygonal playhouse as well as its fame and influence – Shakespeare almost certainly started his London career here. Much of its history is also preserved in numerous legal cases. The Curtain, owned at one time by Henry Laneman, is known to have been transformed into tenements by the 1640s and it was still standing many years later, making it the longest surviving of all the London playhouses.

London's theatre district shifted southwards to the Bankside, already known for various unsavoury entertainments, with the construction of the Rose in 1587. The discovery of the Rose (1587) during a routine rescue dig in 1989 was a milestone in what has become 'Shakespearean archaeology'. The historical importance of the Rose lay in the survival of extensive papers belonging to its owner Philip Henslowe, now in Dulwich College. Of the sites investigated, it has been the largest excavation by far, thus producing more information than the others. The Theatre, Curtain and Rose all appeared to be the same size and shape – albeit further developed during their lifetimes – but the next Bankside playhouse, the 1595 Swan, was larger. Its location a little farther upstream is known from contemporary maps but any archaeological remains are assumed to be destroyed by extensive and deep basements covering the site. The Globe was built in 1599 by Burbage's sons along with five others including William Shakespeare, as a successor to the Theatre just 100m south-east of the Rose. It has been made the most famous of the London playhouses through its association with Shakespeare, but it does not have as much documented history as many of the others and though the north-eastern part of the building was excavated in 1989, only limited information was retrieved. The Rose and the Globe excavations were published fully in 2009 (Bowsher and Miller 2009).

There was another shift to the north when the Fortune was built in Cripplegate in 1600. This was another Henslowe enterprise and its size and location is known largely through the survival of its building contract and other documents. From these, we learn that it was to be based on the Globe, and built by the same carpenter, but was square in shape. Henslowe returned to the south bank for the last of the playhouses, the Hope, which is also well known through his papers which revealed that it was to be based on the Swan. Innovative as ever, Henslowe had the Hope designed as a dual purpose building; having a removable stage allowing for animal baiting for half the week. After only a few years the actors left in dissatisfaction and the venue remained a 'beargarden' until its demolition in 1656. A small area was excavated between 1999 and 2001 and only recently published, as a chapter in a larger account of excavations in the area (Mackinder et al. 2013).

The taphouses

These playhouses had their main entrance on the nearest thoroughfare for easy public access and the stage will have been opposite. Their form is well known today from the reconstructed Globe on the south bank of the Thames: a simple ring of galleries providing three tiers of (probably) seated accommodation around a yard open to the skies wherein the 'groundlings' stood to watch the plays performed on a stage that projected into this yard. The area behind the stage was known as the 'tiring house' from actors attiring but it must have also housed a variety of 'management' offices. However, there was no room for any internal services – a bar or a foyer, let alone conveniences – in the modern sense. Provision, therefore, was made through the dedicated 'taphouses' attached to most of them. It might be assumed however, that at the two inns, the Boar's Head in Whitechapel and the Red Bull in Clerkenwell, that were permanently transformed into playhouses (in 1598 and 1607), might have continued the provisioning of the former businesses for their new clientele. Such may also have been the case at the short lived Red Lion, said to have been built near or next to a farm, which might have supplied seasonal victualling. The Newington Butts plot appears to have had two buildings on it and that not used as a playhouse may have doubled as Savage's dwelling and as a taphouse (Ingram 1971, 388, 389, 392; Ingram 1992, 150–181).

There is no mention of a taphouse next to the Theatre, though the lease included other buildings on its eastern side that could have been used as such. The grounds of the former Priory of Holywell certainly had bakehouses and brewhouses as part of the usual service buildings associated with such an establishment. Indeed, the Survey of London's 'conjectural plan' locates one of the bakehouses in the area of the Theatre (Bird and Norman 1922, 170, Pl83), and an oven found in the excavations very much predated the construction of the Theatre. Just to the south of the playhouse was a 'great barn' which by 1576 had been made into two tenements, one of which was occupied by Hugh Richards, an innholder, though which inn and where is not known (Wickham et al. 2000, 133; Bowsher 2007). It had been suggested that when Burbage lived in Coleman Street (before moving to Shoreditch in 1576) he might have known Richards who would have been a neighbour. Thus it was speculated that Richards might have told Burbage about the availability of land – to build a playhouse – and 'might have seen some advantage to himself in the nearby presence of a playing place' (Ingram 1992, 185). However, it appears that Burbage decided to manage any provisioning himself. In June 1581 he was fined for keeping an unlicenced 'tippling house' in Holywell Street – where he lived and which might even have been an adjunct to his own house – from which he sold food and drink to playgoers. He continued to be indicted up to 1595 which suggests that not only was he persistently offending but that playgoers were still being successfully provided for, off premises (Eccles, 1991, 43).

The public house now known as the Horse and Groom, on the Curtain Street frontage near the assumed entrance to the Curtain Playhouse, appears to be the latest (1890s) manifestation in a long line of taverns or inns going back to the eighteenth century at least. In 1598 Everard Guilpin's satire of the citizen 'who, coming from the Curtain, sneaketh in to some odd garden noted house of sin' (Wickham et al. 2000, 412) may allow us to speculate that an adjacent establishment offered a variety of refreshments. Burbage and Brayne's dealings with Laneman has suggested that by 1592 they had bought the Curtain as an 'easer' to the Theatre (discussed in full in Ingram 1992, 227–236). Nevertheless, Burbage's nearby tippling house may have provided for the audience at the Curtain too.

The first playhouse whose catering facilities that we have written evidence for was the Rose. The earliest document to give details of the building of the playhouse, the so called 'partnership agreement' of January 1587 between Henslowe and John Cholmley, is in fact a curious financial deal (Ingram 2012) but it also contains what would be called a 'catering franchise' today (Bowsher and Cerasano 2009). Henslowe had taken the lease on a large piece of ground in 1585 and in 1587 hived off the southern portion for the new playhouse enterprise. In the south-west corner of this plot, fronting Maid Lane (now Park Street) there was an existing building – 'that small tenement or dwelling house situated and standing at the south end or side of the said parcel of ground or garden plot' in which we assume Cholmley was the sitting tenant. The agreement then notes that the house was 'to keep victualing in or to put to any other use or uses whatsoever with the whole benefit, proffit & commodity which he the said John Cholmley his executors or assignes shall or may receive or make of'. Cholmley was to have exclusive right to the catering and victualling of the enterprise run from his house.

This building was found in the excavations and we suggest that alterations to it may have been connected to the construction of the larger playhouse immediately to the east and north-east of it This house was fairly small and its most likely use was for the storage, and thus distribution, of foodstuffs and drink, although again its size would limit large quantities of material. Regrettably, there was little information from the building, in botanical or artefactual remains, that might have aided an identification of usage within it (Bowsher and Miller 2009, 28–32).

What might have been the first purpose-built taphouse is the small building seen just behind, to the west of, the Swan on a plan of 1627 (Foakes 1985, 24–25), though there is no documentary evidence for such an establishment. The Globe was built only four years after the Swan and may have been the same size as it. Here, there is explicit documentary evidence for a taphouse built by one of the shareholders, John Hemminges. It was burnt down, along with the Globe itself in June 1613, but was rebuilt in 1614 (Egan 2001). Wenceslaus Hollar's drawing of Bankside shows a small building at the back of the Globe that must surely be that taphouse (Foakes 1985, 29–30, 36–38), in exactly the same relation to the Globe playhouse as the earlier small building was to the Swan. Limited excavations on the playhouse site did not extend to the area of the tap-house (Bowsher and Miller 2009, 86–107).

Philip Henslowe's ultimate heir, the actor Edward Alleyn, leased out the Fortune playhouse property to the resident playing company in October 1618, which included an adjacent taphouse occupied by one Mark Brigham (Greg 1907, 28, 29; Chambers 1923, iii, 442). It was later described as 'belonging' to the playhouse (Bentley 1968, 141). There is no evidence where this taphouse was situated or whether it was an existing building, perhaps on the Golden Lane frontage, or a purpose-built establishment.

There is no mention of any taphouse at the Hope, but we might note that the older bear-garden pulled down in 1614 to make way for it had been furnished with a new gatehouse in 1606, situated on Bankside to the north – from where its entrance clearly lay. Analysis of its building contract strongly suggests that it also functioned as a taphouse (Lawrence and Godfrey 1920, 155) and it seems highly likely that this building, later known as the Dancing Bears tavern, was probably used to serve the Hope in a similar fashion. We might also note that Samuel Pepys recorded an ale-house actually attached to the Davies bear-garden, the last of the Bankside animal arenas just to the south of the earlier Hope. Excavations there revealed a larger area on the northern side of the building that has been identified with Pepys' ale-house (Saxby forthcoming).

The use of an existing building adjacent to a playhouse was obviously attractive and sales of 'victuals' may have offset the loss of rental income. It is also likely that the playhouses needed further areas of storage for costumes and props than could be found in the backstage areas. A new building however, could be sited for maximum provision, sale and even storage.

At the Rose, Cholmey was allowed to present his victualling for 'sale in or about the saide parcel of ground, playhouse or garden plot and other the premises' which would encompass the entire site. There was not a lot of space around the Rose and playgoers may have queued up at Cholmley's front door on Maid Lane to obtain victualling before going into the playhouse, again via Maid Lane. Similarly sited buildings on the road front near or next to the playhouse entrances may also have occurred at the Theatre, Curtain and Fortune. At the Hope, provision was probably made from an existing building, but one that had served the same function earlier.

Alternatively at the Rose, staff may have transported victuals straight into the playhouse via a back door, or 'stage door' or as must be the case here; a 'service entrance'. There was certainly a 'tiring house door' at the Rose after its alterations in 1592, and perhaps earlier, and probably one recorded at the Globe in 1613 (Bowsher and Miller 2009, 114). In 1599 Thomas Platter noted that 'during the performance food and drink are carried around the audience, so that for what one cares to pay one may also have refreshment' (translation in Chambers 1923, ii, 365). In 1614 Thomas Overbury described 'a Water-bearer on the floor of a play-house' (Gurr 2004, 273), perhaps carrying the 'peculiar wooden vessels' used by London water sellers noted by Jacob Rathgeb in 1592 (Porter 2009, 96). The playhouse water seller may have been one of the taphouse staff or an independent entrepreneur. The former is more likely as at the Rose, Cholmley was given exclusive rights within the entire site. Nevertheless, the mechanism and route by which victuals were transported through a back door then perhaps into the galleries and then down into the yard is poorly understood and has not been solved by archaeology. What archaeology has provided is direct evidence for vessels used within the playhouses and foodstuffs themselves.

The vessels

Vessels are absent from the list of props that Henslowe had at the Rose (Foakes 2002, 316–25) but they must have been used. Bowls, dishes and cups were the most common props referred to in the numerous 'banqueting scenes' in plays of the time (Meads 2001, 50).

The pottery assemblage from the Rose, Globe and Theatre excavations, stratigraphically associated with playhouse use, was largely made in post-medieval redwares, mostly London and Surrey-Hampshire border ware. There was a high proportion of 'cooking vessels' such as cauldrons, tripod pipkins, skillets, bowls, colanders and chafing dishes, and flanged or flared dishes and porringers, which were almost certainly used for 'serving'. The next highest category of pottery came from drinking – or drink serving – vessels. These included drinking jugs, tygs, tankards, mugs and a Border whiteware pedestal goblet from the Theatre (illustrated in Bowsher 2012, 191), though it is not possible to know whether they contained beer/ale or even wine.

There are no vessels which could be said to be of high status, though there were a number of imported decorated Bartmann jugs, most are very typical domestic household vessels. They may have been brought into the playhouse from the taphouses or by the audience (Bowsher and Miller 2009, 147–8, 153). Fragments of an exceptional Surrey-Hampshire border ware jug with anthropomorphic medallions (reminiscent of the typical 'Shakespeare image'), however, were found in demolition deposits at the Theatre (Knight 2009, 349).

In contrast, the assemblage of glassware vessels from similar deposits at the Rose (very little was found at the Globe or Theatre) is unusual overall in including several fragments from vessels/lids which are considered very high-status items, as well as more commonly encountered ones. A jar and the three relatively early lids are rare, and a pedestal beaker is very rare. The vessels are mainly either green (i.e. potash glass, probably made in England) or colourless (the more prestigious soda glass, which may have been imported from Venice or Antwerp).

The storage bottles are routine vessels, but, like the flask, their presence, along with the varied serving wares, may be seen as a reflection of refreshments sold at the taphouse as much (particularly with the more prestigious wares) as drinks brought in by the audience from nearby taverns or from home. The three lids could have been used to help contain drinks brought some distance on foot.

The ceramic drinking vessels were found throughout the Rose site, though there was a respectable number below the galleries but only a few below the first stage. There was a large collection of all types, however, in the dumps over the first stage and in the floor of the second. Interestingly, there was also a concentration of the higher status glass drinking vessels associated with the second stage area. The preponderance of 'banqueting scenes' in contemporary drama might also explain the proportion of such vessels in the stage area, as might the backstage festivities of actors and wealthier patrons.

Finally it should be noted that a pewter tankard lid, from a late demolition fill, may originally have been associated either with a glass or a fine ceramic vessel. At the other end of the market, the base of a wooden tankard was found in the sealing deposits covering the Rose playhouse remains (Bowsher and Miller 2009, 152–3). Apart from the 'water' being carried around, the only clear reference to what was actually being drunk at the playhouses is to 'bottled ale'. This liquid was used to extinguish the burning breeches of the unfortunate man caught up in the Globe fire in June 1613 (Chambers 1923 ii, 419). According to Thomas Stephens, writing in 1615, the sound of bottled ale being opened at the theatre or playhouse was a common distraction (Gurr 2004a, 43).

A few items of cutlery were found at the Rose excavations and it is tempting to associate a broken pewter spoon with the initials AE with the actor Edward Alleyn – the 'star' of the Rose. It certainly dates to the late sixteenth/early seventeenth century but was found in post-playhouse dumps (Bowsher and Miller 2009, 211). Much more prestigious was a very high quality 'sucket fork' possibly of Netherlandish origin, generally used for sweetmeats, found in dumps over the stage. It represents an early use of the fork, hitherto associated with advanced continental dining (MacGregor 2012, 32–33) and may reflect ostentatious consumption at the playhouse (Bowsher and Miller 2009, 212; Bate and Thornton 2012, 46).

Foodstuffs

Contemporary 'dietaries' and textual studies (Fitzpatrick 2007) provide a large body of evidence as to what sort of food was eaten by Londoners in the late sixteenth/early seventeenth century (note also Porter 2009, Chapter 4). Nevertheless, virtually anything was available to the rich, as noted in William Harrison's 1577 chapter on the 'Of the food and diet of the English' (Harrison 2001). The Henslowe–Cholmley agreement of 1587 notes that the latter had for sale 'any bread or drink' at the Rose, corroborated by Platter's account of 'food and drink'. Paul Hentzner, visiting London in 1598, recorded that at the playhouses 'fruits, such as apples, pears and nuts, according to the season, are carried about to be sold, as well as wine and ale' (Chambers 1923, II 363 for the original Latin; Rye 1865, 216 for an English translation).

This is supported to some degree by the archaeobotanical evidence from the Rose excavations. Whilst wild fruit seeds found at the Rose were probably related to the local environment such seeds found below the audience galleries are more likely to have been consumption waste. Although apples are mentioned in contemporary accounts, their seeds were not as common within the botanical assemblage of the site as grape, fig, elder, plum and blackberry/raspberry along with pear, cherry and peach found at the Rose, as well as at the Globe. A lot of fruit was imported into London in the sixteenth century and dried fruit such as raisins, currants, prunes, figs and dates were popular at the time (Porter 2009, 93). An interesting component within the food remains, were numerous *Cucurbitaceae* (marrow/pumpkin, squash/gourd) seeds as they represent relatively early evidence of contact with the New World (Bowsher and Miller 2009, 149–50).

Within the historical records, there are also references to 'sweetmeats', liquorice, green ginger and sugar-candy (Chambers 1923 II, 548 & n7). Lines from *Wit Without Money* of *c*. 1614, refer to apprentices at the theatre/playhouse cracking nuts (Chambers 1923 II, 533 n2), a phrase later made famous as theatre/playhouse attendance generally by Lawrence (1935). There were walnut and hazel shells at the Rose, though most of the latter was waste from soap manufacture and here used constructionally, as a conglomerate floor surface (Orrell, 1992; Bowsher and Miller 2009, 61).

There is limited evidence from the other playhouse excavation sites, but charred cereal grain was found in the demolition deposits of the Theatre in Shoreditch. Aside from the archaeobotanical evidence, animal bones found at the Rose and other contemporary sites largely relate to post playhouse dumps of waste rather than *in situ* consumption waste. The assemblage was dominated by sheep/goat and, to a lesser extent, cattle and pig with smaller amounts of chicken, fish (mostly herring and eel), and rabbit. Such a range is fairly uniform on most contemporary sites. Higher status meat was represented by deer and sparrow/lark bones but the carapace of a green turtle and two fragments from a bear paw/foot may confer a unique culinary presence on the Rose estate, or at least its immediate environs. If these represent food waste they are certainly rare delicacies. The turtle remains are only the second found from London and bears' feet were specifically described as 'the best morsel' in 1576 (Reilly in Bowsher and Miller 2009, 248–52). Nevertheless, numerous larger bear bones, along with dog and horse bones, were found in dumps at the Rose and other Bankside sites that must have been waste from the nearby animal-baiting arenas. Some of these have butchering and teeth marks indicating that they were fed to the surviving dog packs kept at these establishments.

By far the largest amount of invertebrate foodstuffs from the Rose playhouse (and post-playhouse) deposits was of common oysters. Good, large oysters were recorded as being common in London in 1592 (Porter 2009, 93) and the plethora found at the Rose (and most contemporary sites) contributed to the media interest in 'Shakespearean snack food' (for example, Keys 2010). Nevertheless, these were supplemented by cockle, mussel, a few periwinkles and whelks; more exotic were the fragments of cuttlefish and edible crab. Taken together therefore, the archaeological and historical evidence demonstrates that a variety of foodstuffs, chiefly fruits, nuts and seafood, were consumed within the theatres themselves, allowing us perhaps to be able to draw distinctions between snacks and the meals consumed in domestic contexts across the city.

Conclusions

Review of the documentary sources in the light of archaeological excavation and research has presented a pattern of playhouse provisioning. The known taphouses do not appear to be very big and it is unlikely that they housed brewing or cooking facilities on a large-enough scale. This was a period when brewing was becoming a specialized commercial operation and supplies to the smaller inns and taphouses would be brought in rather than brewed on the premises (cf Carlin 1996, Chapter 8; Clark 1983, 115). It was also a period when many houses did not have an oven, and pies and the like would be taken down to the local bakery for cooking (Picard 2003, 174–5). It is likely that these taphouses were just used for storage and dissemination. That dissemination may have involved playgoers queuing at a counter as well as provisions being carried around the auditorium, perhaps dependant on where the building was in relation to the playhouse.

Taken together therefore, the archaeological and historical evidence demonstrates that a variety of foodstuffs, chiefly fruits, nuts and seafood, were consumed within the playhouses themselves, allowing us perhaps to be able to draw distinctions between theatrical snacks and the meals consumed in domestic contexts across the city. Nevertheless, Shakespearean snacks appear to have been healthier than the G and T and crisps in our modern theatres.

Acknowledgements

I am grateful to the organizers of the Exeter conference for inviting me to speak on what was one of the most modern of the archaeological topics. The first part of this paper concerns food provision within the various playhouse venues, some of it new research. Much of the second part, based on actual remains found at the Rose and Globe Theatre, rests on the work done by many specialist colleagues to whom I am indebted: Lucy Whittingham (pottery), the late Geoff Egan (glass), Kevin Reilly (animal bone), John Giorgi (botanical remains) and Alan Pipe (invertebrates). Last but not least, I am grateful to my colleagues Pat Miller (co-author of the Rose and the Globe publication, responsible for the Globe) and Heather Knight (who supervised the recent excavations at the Theatre and Curtain) for comments on this paper.

References

Angus, J. 1862. *The works of Thomas Adams: The sum of his sermons, meditations, and other divine and moral meditations, Vol. II*, Edinburgh.
Bate, J. and Thornton, D. 2012. *Shakespeare: staging the world*, London.
Bentley, G.E. 1968. *The Jacobean and Caroline stage, Vol 6*, Oxford.
Bowsher, J.M.C. 2011. 'Twenty years on: The archaeology of 'Shakespeare's' London playhouses', *Shakespeare, Journal of the British Shakespeare Association* 7(4), 452–466.
Bowsher, J.M.C. 2012. *Shakespeare's London Theatreland; archaeology, history drama*, London.
Bowsher, J.M.C. and Cerasano, S.P. 2009. 'The Deed of Partnership in the Rose Playhouse (January 10, 1587)'. Henslowe-Alleyn Digital Project; Digital Essay: http://www.henslowe-alleyn.org.uk/essays/rosecontract.html
Bowsher, J.M.C. and Miller, P. 2009. *The Rose and the Globe – playhouses of Shakespeare's Bankside: excavations 1989–1991*, Museum of London Archaeology Monograph 48, London.
Bird, J. and Norman, P. (eds.), 1922. *Survey of London. Vol VIII; The parish of St Leonard, Shoreditch*, London.
Chambers, E.K. 1923. *The Elizabethan Stage*, 4 vols, Oxford.

Clark, P. 1983. *The English alehouse; a social history 1200–1830*, London.
Dessen, A.C. and Thomson, L. 1999. *A Dictionary of Stage Directions in English Drama, 1580–1642*, Cambridge.
Eccles, M. 1991. 'Elizabethan actors I: A–D', *Notes & Queries* 236/1, 38–49.
Egan, G. 2001. 'John Hemminges's Tap-house at the Globe', *Theatre Notebook* 55, 72–77.
Fitzpatrick, J. 2007. *Food in Shakespeare: Early modern dietaries and the plays*, Farnham.
Foakes, R.A. 1985. *Illustrations of the English stage 1580–1642*, London.
Greg, W.W. (ed.) 1907. *Henslowe papers, being documents supplementary to Henslowe's diary*, 2 vols, London.
Gurr, A. 2004. *Playgoing in Shakespeare's London*, (3rd edition), Cambridge.
Harrison, W. 1577. *A description of Elizabethan England; Chapter VI. Of the food and diet of the English*. Harvard Classics, Vol 35, Part 3, New York, 2001 http://www.bartleby.com/35/3/6.html
Ingram, W. 1971. 'The playhouse at Newington Butts: A new proposal', *Shakespeare Quarterly* 21, 385–98.
Ingram, W. 1992. *The business of playing: The beginnings of the adult professional theatre in Elizabethan London*, Ithaca and London.
Ingram, W. 2012. 'John Chomley on the Bankside', *Early Theatre* 15(2), 43–66.
Keys, D. 2010. 'Fancy oysters with your Shakespeare ?' *The Independent*, Friday 29 January 2010, p.17 http://www.independent.co.uk/arts-entertainment/theatre-dance/news/fancy-oysters-with-your-shakespeare-1882563.html
Knight, H. 2009. 'Shakespeare's Theatre? Excavations at 4–6 New Inn Broadway, London EC2', *Post-Medieval Archaeology* 43(2), 347–349.
Lawrence, J. and Godfrey, W.H. 1920. 'The Bear-Garden Contract of 1606 and what it implies', *Architectural Review* xlvii, 152–5.
Lawrence, W.J. 1935. *Those nut-cracking Elizabethans: Studies of the early theatre and drama*, London.
Mackinder, A. with Blackmore, L., Bowsher, J.C. and Phillpotts, C. 2013. *The Hope playhouse, animal baiting and later industrial activity at Bear Gardens on Bankside: excavations at Riverside House and New Globe Walk, Southwark, 1999–2000*. MOLA Archaeology Studies Series 25, London.
MacGregor, N. 2012. *Shakespeare's restless world*, London.
Meads, C. 2001. *Banquets set forth: banqueting in English Renaissance drama*, Manchester.
Orrell, J. 1992. 'Nutshells at the Rose', *Theatre Research International* 17, 8–14.
Picard, L. 2003. *Elizabeth's London: Everyday life in Elizabethan London*, London.
Porter, S. 2009. *Shakespeare's London; everyday life in London 1580–1616*, Stroud.
Rye, W.B. 1865. *England as seen by foreigners, in the days of Elizabeth & James the first*, London (reprinted New York 1967).
Saxby, D. Forthcoming. "A very rude and nasty pleasure'; Davies' Bear Garden, Bankside, Southwark'. *Surrey Archaeological Collections*.
Wallace, C.W. 1913. *The first London theatre: materials for a history*, Nebraska.
Wickham, G., Berry, H. and Ingram, W. 2000. *English Professional Theatre, 1530–1660*, Cambridge.

What Shall We Grow? Continuity and Change in Prehistoric Farming in Croatia and Serbia.

Kelly Reed
University of Leicester

This short paper summarizes on-going research on archaeobotanical remains collected from 18 sites within Croatia and Serbia, ranging from the Late Neolithic to the Late Bronze Age (5500–800 BC). The archaeobotanical remains allow us to look at the decisions made by local farming communities to cultivate, introduce, or to cease cultivating certain crop species. From the Late Neolithic through to the Late Bronze Age we see the occurrence of many socio-cultural and economic changes in south-east European societies, such as the introduction of metallurgy, the growth of trade, and evidence for increasing centralization of power. Agriculture would have been central to everyday life at this time, and as such must have both underpinned these developments and been changed by them. This project is an investigation into the way people lived and how changes in settlement, burial and technology impacted on the way food was grown and how food production may have shaped these changes.

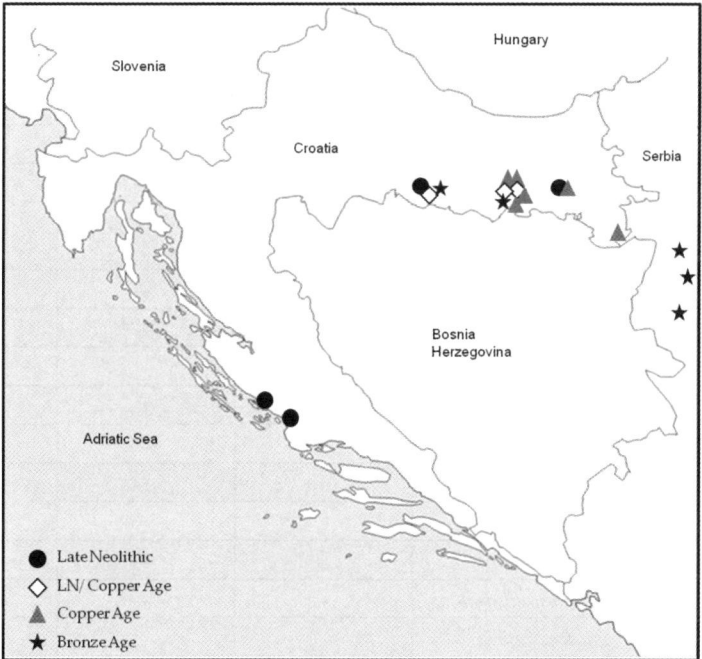

Figure 11.1. Site locations within Croatia and Serbia.

What were they growing?

Between 2006 and 2010 archaeobotanical material was collected from 15 sites across Croatia (Figure 11.1). Four are Late Neolithic sites (*c.* 5500–4500 BC), three span the Late Neolithic/Copper Age (*c.* 5000–4000 BC), six are Copper Age sites (*c.* 4500–2700 BC), and two are dated to the Bronze Age (*c.* 2700–800 BC). All samples were recovered from archaeological structures related to human activities, i.e. settlement areas such as house floors, pits, and ditches. In addition to this, three published Bronze Age sites located in north-west Serbia were also selected for future detailed statistical analysis, Gomolava, Feudvar and Židovar (Kroll 1998; Medović 2002; van Zeist 2003).

The type of strategy adopted by a farmer will depend on a number of local circumstances, such as the availability of land, labour and tools (technology), and the socio-economic climate (for example, population pressures and the opportunity to trade). In addition, the farmer has to consider which crops to grow based on whether manure is available (for example, considering pastoral regimes) and the local environment (for example, temperature, topography, and soil conditions). All these factors will dictate the types of regimes that could be employed. Preliminary results seen in Table 11.1 show the relative abundance of crop remains recovered from all 18 sites for each period.

Table 11.1. Relative abundance of crop remains recovered from 18 sites within Croatia and Serbia (+ sporadic; ++ little; +++ abundant).

Taxon		Late Neolithic	Copper Age	Bronze Age
Barley	(*Hordeum vulgare*)	+	+++	+++
Einkorn	(*Triticum monococcum*)	+++	+++	+++
Emmer	(*Triticum dicoccum*)	+++	+++	+++
Free-threshing wheat	(*T. aestivum/durum*)	+	++	+++
Spelt	(*Triticum spelta*)	+	+	++
Broomcorn millet	(*Panicum miliaceum*)	+	++	+++
Grass pea	(*Lathyrus sativus*)	+	+	+++
Lentil	(*Lens culinaris*)	++	+	+++
Pea	(*Pisum sativum*)	+	+	++
Bitter vetch	(*Vicia ervilia*)	+	+	++
Broad bean	(*Vicia faba*)	-	-	+
Chickpea	(*Cicer arietinum*)	-	-	+
Flax	(*Linum usitatissimum*)	+	-	++
Gold of pleasure	(*Camelina sativa*)	-	-	+++

Plant remains from the Late Neolithic indicate a dominance of einkorn and emmer wheat with a very narrow range of other crops. During the Copper Age there is evidence of the continued use of emmer and einkorn with increased presence of barley, free-threshing wheat and millet. By the Bronze Age, we can see that agricultural diversity seems to increase with a greater variety of crops present in the assemblages. During this period a number of new species begin to be utilized by farmers including chickpea, broad bean and gold of pleasure, a plant used for its oil. The use of the plough, from the Copper Age, would have significantly increased the agricultural potential of lands allowing a variety of growing conditions to be exploited (Halstead 1995; Sherratt 1981). The introduction of new technology (for example, metallurgy, wheel, plough) and new species (for example, chickpea, gold of pleasure) would have provided the farmer with the opportunity to grow a greater variety of crops.

Continuity or change?

The preliminary results show a continuation in the cultivation of emmer and einkorn from the Late Neolithic through to the Late Bronze Age. The emergence of new crops during the later periods, most notably the Bronze Age, indicates an increase in diversification by the farming communities in this region. By examining not only the archaeobotanical data but also the archaeological context a more cohesive interpretation of the agricultural regimes employed will be possible. Further research will explore the social and economic changes within this region and how these interlink with the archaeobotanical evidence. For example, settlement patterns in south-east Europe change from large tell sites in the Late Neolithic, to small dispersed farms in the Copper Age, and to a mixture of large tell and small farm settlements in the Bronze Age. Thus, by examining the archaeobotanical evidence it may be possible to explore whether farming practices influenced changes in settlement patterns or adapted to them.

Acknowledgements

I wish to thank Jacqueline Balen at the Museum of Zagreb, Maja Krznarić Škrivanko and Hrvoje Vulic from Vinkovci Museum, Emil Podrug from Sibenik Museum, Marija Mihaljević from Nova Gradiška Museum and Helmut Kroll at the University of Kiel for allowing me to use their material and for all their help over the years. Thanks to my proof readers, my supervisor Prof van der Veen and to AHRC for their financial support.

References

Halstead, P. 1995. 'Plough and power: the economic and social significance of cultivation with the ox-drawn ard in the Mediterranean', *Bulletin on Sumerian Agriculture* 8, 11–22.

Kroll, H. 1998. 'Die Kultur- und Naturland- schaften des Titeler Plateaus im Spiegel der metall- zeitlichen Pflanzenreste von Feudvar – Biljni svet Teitelskog platoa u bronzanum i gvozdenom dobu –

Palaeobotanička analiza biljnih ostataka praistorijskog naselja Feudvar', in Hänsel, B. and Medović, P. (eds.), *Feudvar 1. Das Plateau von Titel und die Šajkaška* (Prähistorische Archäologie in Südosteuropa 13), Kiel, 305–317.

Medović, A. 2002. 'Arheobotanička istraživanja metalodobnog naselja Židovar, Vojvodina/Jugoslavija – preliminarni izveštaj', *СТАРИНАР (Starinar)* 52, 181–190.

Sherratt, A. 1981. 'Plough and pastoralism: aspects of the secondary products revolution', in Hodder, I., Isaac, G. and Hammond, N. (eds.), *Pattern of the Past,* Cambridge, 261–301.

van Zeist, W. 2003. 'Plant husbandry and vegetation of tell Gomolava, Vojvodina, Yugoslavia', *Palaeohistoria* 43/44, 87–115.

The Processing and Treatment of Drinking Water in Iberia (c. Sixth–Second Centuries BC)

Meritxell Oliach Fàbregas
Institut Català d'Arqueologia Clàssica

This paper illustrates the different solutions used by protohistoric communities for the catchment, storage, and conservation of water. I will particularly focus on the processing of water for human consumption during the Iberian period in the far north-east of the Iberian zone (present-day Catalonia, southern France and eastern Aragon).

The available archaeological data, as well as the ethnographic research, have enabled me to further develop my research into water in protohistory. My previous work consisted of an initial compilation of the different processes and treatments received by water before its consumption. Now I begin to outline the levels of quality and salubrity in the Iberian period. Finally, this research has shown that the process undergone by water from its catchment to its consumption was more complex than I had originally thought.

The aim of this paper is to put together the first compilation of documents and information on the different urban water management solutions used during the protohistory of the north-eastern Iberian Peninsula. I also intend to analyse the protohistoric water supply structures in the above-mentioned area on a morphological, spatial and functional level. By examining the archaeological data, and through ethnographic parallels, I will evaluate the possible water extraction, treatment and usage systems, as well as the utility of the water supply structures and their significance within the context of Iberian society.

Structures for collecting water
The documented water catchment structures include containers or large vessels, springs, pond-cisterns and wells. To begin with, amphoras or large jars were placed on the tops of houses or below gutters to collect the rainwater that flowed off the roofs. It is difficult to identify this type of jar among the sherds of common ware; however, examples have been documented *in situ*, including some at Puig Castellar (Santa Coloma de Gramanet, Barcelona) (Ferrer et al. 2003, 31). As for springs, despite their long use as places of worship or for water catchment, we only know of one spring located inside a settlement in the whole of Iberia, at Collado de los Jardines (Santa Elena, Jaén) (Calvo and Cabré 1918 and 1919). However, springs are often located on the access slopes to settlements, some of which were sought out by digging underground galleries or were altered to make it easier to access the water.

Processing and Treatment of Drinking Water in Iberia

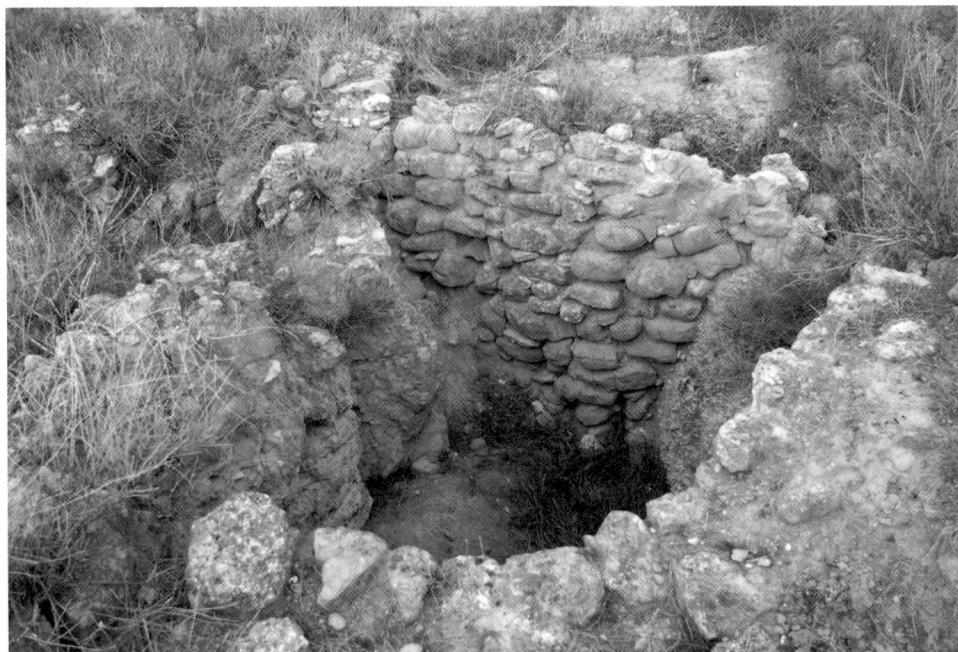

Figure 12.1. Cistern at Tossal de les Tenalles (Sidamón) (Photo: M. Oliach).

The documented ponds or cisterns are underground reservoirs, many of which are partially or totally lined with stones bound together with mud. They normally occupied a central position inside the settlement and were closely related to the layout of the road network. The earliest pond/cistern found on the Iberian Peninsula is that of Fuente Álamo (Cuevas de Almanzora, Almería), dating from the end of the second millennium BC (Schubart et al. 2000).

In the north-eastern area, the earliest examples of this solution are found in Aragon, the oldest of them being the first cistern of Zafranales (Fraga) (Montón 2000), which was built in the Late Bronze Age (*c.* 1100 BC). In Catalonia, the first example is at Tossal de les Tenalles (Sidamón, Lleida) from the ninth–eighth centuries BC (Marí et al. 1993) (Figure 12.1). In France there are no examples until the second or first centuries BC, when the cisterns of La Cloche (Les Pennes-Mirabeau, Bouches-du-Rhône) (Chabot 1992) and Ensérune (Hérault) (Jannoray 1955) were built.

Finally, there are few known examples of protohistoric wells in the north-eastern Iberian Peninsula. Among the different examples of wells inside an enclosure one could mention those of Alorda Park (Calafell, Tarragona) (Asensio et al. 1996), Palermo I (Casp, Zaragoza) (Pellicer 1952, 395) (this could be Republican), Puig Castellet (Lloret de Mar, Girona) (Pons et al. 1989, 212, 215), and Vilars (Arbeca, Lleida). Others are found at Can Xercavins (Cerdanyola, Barcelona) and Castell de Rubí (Barcelona) (Francès et al. 1995), although we do not know whether they were inside or outside the

Processing and Treatment of Drinking Water in Iberia

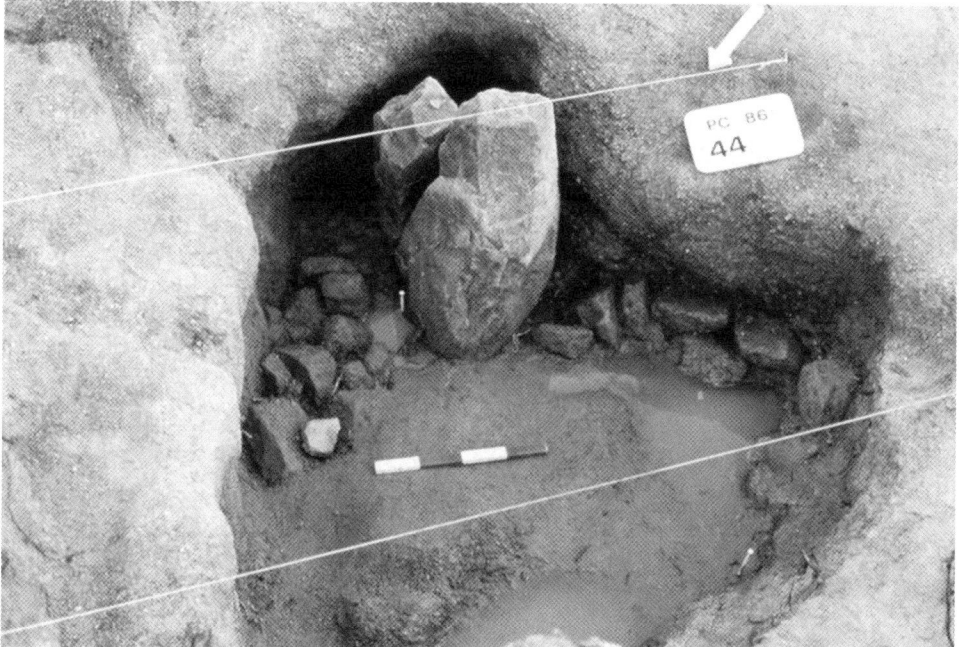

Figure 12.2. Filtration system documented at Puig Castellet (Lloret de Mar) (Pons et al. 1989, 215).

inhabited area. They are wells dug into the ground, many of which are lined with stones bound together with mud and they can be as deep as 11m. They do not appear to have existed before the fifth century BC.

Extracting the water from wells and cisterns

Despite the lack of documentation, I propose the following solutions: the bucket, the *mêntal*, and the chadouf. The use of buckets is evidenced by the marks left by ropes as they rubbed against the sides of the well rims. The method was improved with the use of the pulley from the eighth century BC in Assyria and the fifth century BC in Greece, although this system has not been documented on the Iberian Peninsula.

A second solution is the *mêntal*, a tub or receptacle with several symmetrically placed ropes or handles that allowed the operators to keep it stable while raising the water. Its origin is unknown, but its antiquity and simplicity mean that it could have been used in the protohistoric period.

Finally, the chadouf is a bucket fastened with a rope and lifted by a large lever with a counterweight. This device appears to have originated in the East and Far East in the eighteenth century BC and has been documented in Greece in the second half of the sixth century BC and in China in the fourth century BC. Although exactly the same device may not have been used in our area of study, there is likely to have been a similar tilting mechanism with a counterweight.

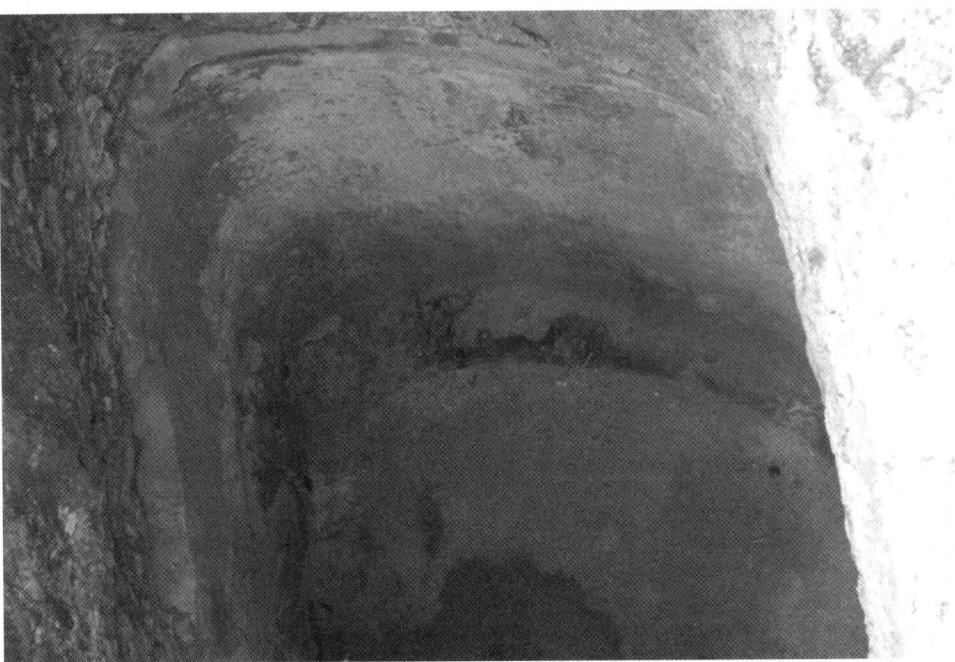

Figure 12.3. Puig de Sant Andreu (Ullastret). Detail of step used for cleaning the cistern (Photo: M. Oliach).

Water processing and treatment

The control of water quality was limited. We have only been able to document hygiene measures of a general nature and processes involving the settling and filtration of the water. Water filtration may have been carried out by depositing branches and twigs in the cistern's adduction channels. This system has been proposed for the small ponds documented along the La Cloche cistern adduction channel (Chabot 1992, 128). A second system was for the water to penetrate through the walls of a first tank into a second, a process that has been documented at Vilars and Puig Castellet, where stones were placed in the first tank for this purpose (Figure 12.2).

In addition, decantation tanks have been documented in front of the storage tanks at the La Cloche and Puig Castellet sites. The accumulated sediment and impurities were removed either via drainage channels or manually. Finally, inside the cisterns there are cleaning and decantation elements, such as pits, cavities and ledges. These have been documented at the La Cloche cistern and in one of those at Sant Andreu d'Ullastret (Girona), in which a small step was used to make cleaning easier (Figure 12.3).

The water could also be treated in other ways before being consumed. It may have been purified by adding salt and certain herbs and boiling or filtering it before it was used for domestic purposes, and we cannot rule out the use of eels or other types of fish to remove mosquito larvae and other remains.

Processing and Treatment of Drinking Water in Iberia

Conclusions

The cistern was used by the Iberians as the main alternative to running water, although the latter must have always been used in preference, as the storage capacity of the cisterns does not appear to be have been sufficient to meet normal needs. Moreover, in many cases, there were no cisterns. Water was extracted manually, as can be seen from the slopes or access ramps to some wells or cisterns. Given the relatively little depth from which the water normally had to be raised, the lifting systems would have been fairly simple and would only have been used sporadically to extract small amounts of water.

The measures taken to ensure the quality of the water were often the same as the general hygiene measures needed for storing it. Many are linked to the building characteristics and particularities of the cisterns, such as their placement below ground to keep the water at a constantly cool temperature and prevent putrefaction, the inclusion of holes cut in the bottom of the cisterns, or a slight slope in the floor of the tank to make it easier to clean the collected water. Filtration mechanisms have also been documented; these used earth, stones or branches, as well as decantation of the water by means of basins and reservoirs linked to the collection and adduction of the water.

According to the information we have, the water from the cisterns would by modern standards have been considered subpotable and drinkable only in case of necessity. Despite the fact that, as we have seen, there was a concern for the salubrity and quality of the water, little was known about pathogens and how to combat them. There was also little knowledge of potability, which would not come until many centuries later, in the industrial era between 1800 and 1950.

Acknowledgements

Supported by the University and Research Commission (Innovation, Universities and Enterprise Department, Generalitat de Catalunya) and the European Social Fund (ESF).

References

Asensio, D., Bruguera, R., Cela, X. and Morer, J. 1996. 'Una mina d'aigua a l'interior de la ciutadella ibèrica d'Alorda Park Calafell, Baix Penedès', *Miscellània Penedesenca* vol. XXIV, 107–144.

Calvo, I. and Cabré, J. 1918 and 1919. *Excavaciones en la cueva y collado de Los Jardines Santa Elena-Jaén*, Memorias de la Junta Superior de excavaciones y Antigüedades, 16 and 22, Madrid.

Chabot, L. 1992. 'La cisterne collective du village de La Cloche, Les Pennes-Mirabeau B.-du-Rh.', *Documents d'Archéologie Méridionale* 15. Protohistoire du sud de la France, 126–130.

Ferrer, C. and Rigo, A. 2003. *Puig Castellar. Els ibers a Santa Coloma. 5 anys d'intervenció arqueològica (1998–2002)*. Monografies locals, 2. Museu Torre Balldovina.

Francès, J. and Carlús, X. 1995. 'Noves dades sobre l'assentament ibèric de Can Xercavins Cerdanyola del Vallès, Vallès Occidental', *Limes* 4–5, 44–61.

Jannoray, J. 1955. *Ensérune, contribution a l'étude des civilisations préromaines de la Gaule Méridionale*. Bibliothèque des Écoles Françaises d'Athènes et de Rome, 181, Paris.

Marí, L., Garcés, I., Pérez, J. and Puche, J.M. 1993. 'Ocupacions de la tradició del Bronze recent i dels camps d'urnes tardans al Tossal de les tenalles de Sidamon', *Revista d'Arqueologia de ponent* 3, Lleida, 249–285.

Montón, F. 2000. 'Zafranales, Fraga, Huesca. Los materiales de la Edad del Bronce', *Bolskan* 17. Huesca, 125–164.

Pellicer, M. 1952. 'Yacimientos arqueológicos en el Término de Caspe', *II Congreso Nacional de Arqueología*, Zaragoza, 389–396.

Pons, E., Llorens, J.M. and Toledo, A. 1989. 'Le hameau fortifié du Puig Castellet à Lloret de Mar Girona, Espagne. Un bilan des recherches', *Documents d'Archéologie Méridionale* 12, 191–222.

Schubart, H., Pingel, V. and Arteaga, O. 2000. *Fuente Álamo. Las excavaciones arqueológicas 1977–1991 en el poblado de la Edad del Bronce*. Arqueología monografías. Junta de Andalucía.

Food Processing and Consumption Spaces: the Case of Molí d'Espígol (Catalonia) in the Third Century BC

Pilar Camañes and Meritxell Monrós
Institut Català d'Arqueologia Clàssica (Rovira i Virgili University, Tarragon)

This paper aims to contribute to the methodology for analysing the spaces used for the preparation and consumption of food (storage, processing and dining spaces) at a specific time during the Iberian period, by defining and studying them at the archaeological site of Molí d'Espígol. Our ultimate objective is to learn more about the organization of each of the stages of the process and the importance given to them by the inhabitants of this site (Figure 13.1). The oldest documented phase, about which we know little, is from the end of the seventh century to the first half of the sixth century BC. The town is characterized by a complex urban planning dating from the fourth century BC, a layout of streets and buildings that survived until the end of the third century BC.

The preparation and storage of food are identified at Molí d'Espígol as complementary activities carried out in the same areas. Each area contained items used for milling, instruments for preparing the raw materials and containers for storing products in large quantities. All this is evidence of a multipurpose use of such spaces. Different tasks, such as milling, the preparation of raw materials using fire and the stockpiling of products, were carried out within these spaces without any apparent direct link to the private or family sphere.

In the evolution of the settlement, this type of space can be clearly seen in Building C. The building covers a total area 18 m long by 10 m wide, encompassing eight different sectors: 15, 17, 19 and 20 in the northern part and 10, 18/26, 24 and 26 on the southern side. The phase we know most about is the third century BC in the southern parts. The most interesting feature of its interior is the paved floor, which was used for grinding and milling and as a hearth, and, to a lesser extent, the benches. Pottery finds consist of high percentages of storage vessels (local and imported amphoras, *kalatos* and jars) and a range of tableware and cooking artefacts (Figure 13.2).

Building A dates from the end of the fourth century BC and survived until the second half of the third century BC. It is made up of various sectors. Building A should be understood as a complex building made up of seven sectors. It was an aristocratic residence in which Room 61 stands out from the rest, both for its size and the finds made in it. In the first half of the third century BC, Sector 61 was used as a meeting area. A large hearth was documented here, as well as many finds, including tableware, serving objects and abundant remains of fauna (ovicaprids, swine and bovines) that had been eaten (Figure 13.3).

Food Processing and Consumption Spaces

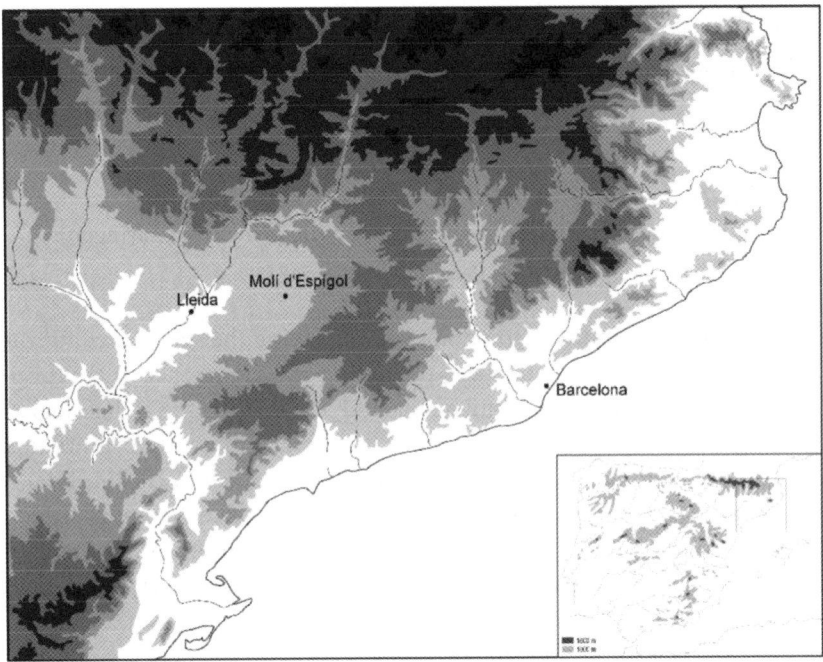

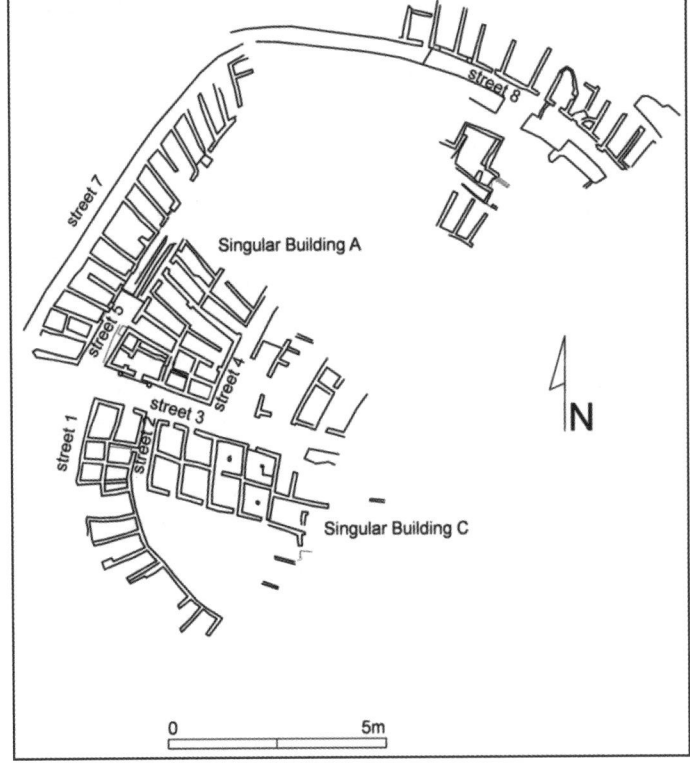

Figure 13.1. Geographical location of the archaeological site (above), and the general plan (left) (P. Camañes and M. Monrós).

Food Processing and Consumption Spaces

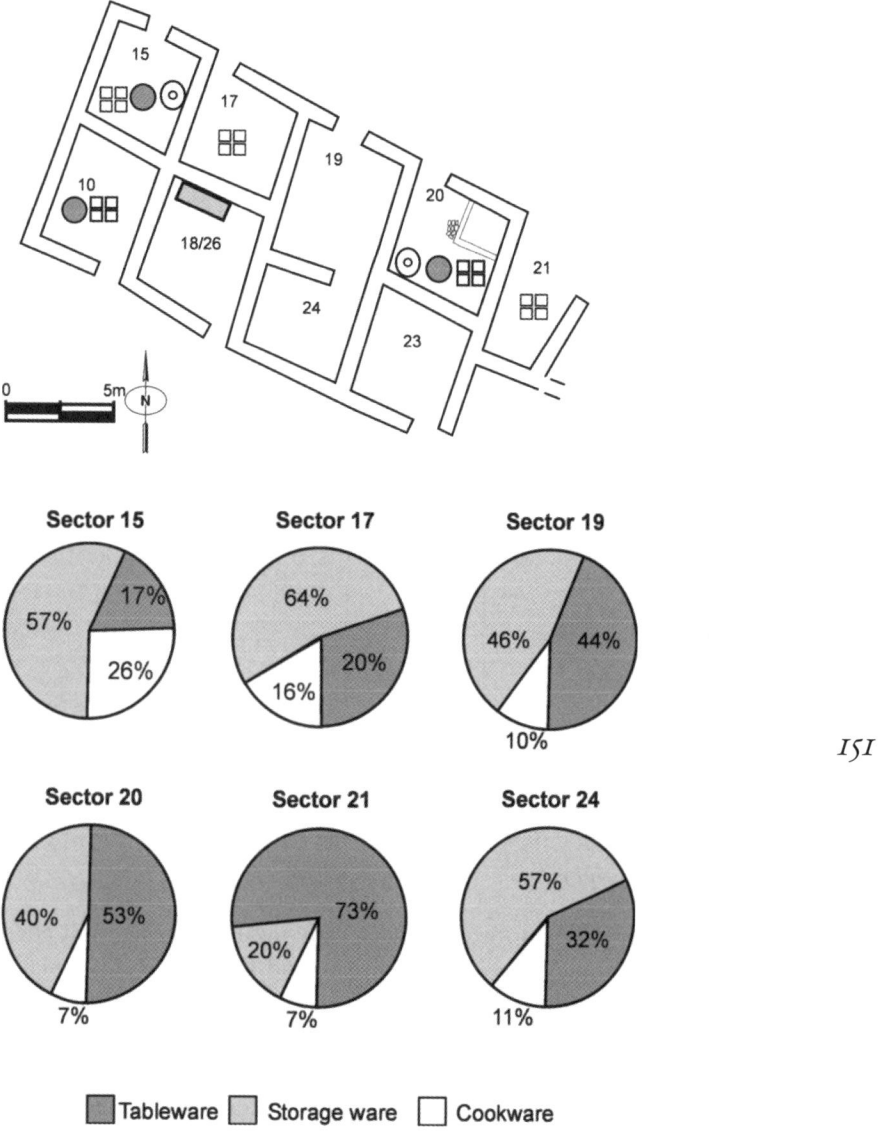

Figure 13.2. Singular Building C plan (top) and graphics quantifying the materials found (below) (P. Camañes).

The central room of the residence was possibly a meeting area in which banquets were held. These would have been *patron-rôle feasts* according to the typology defined by Dietler (1999, 144). The purpose of these would have been to consume massive amounts of food and drink and to strengthen ties between the patron or chief and the client.

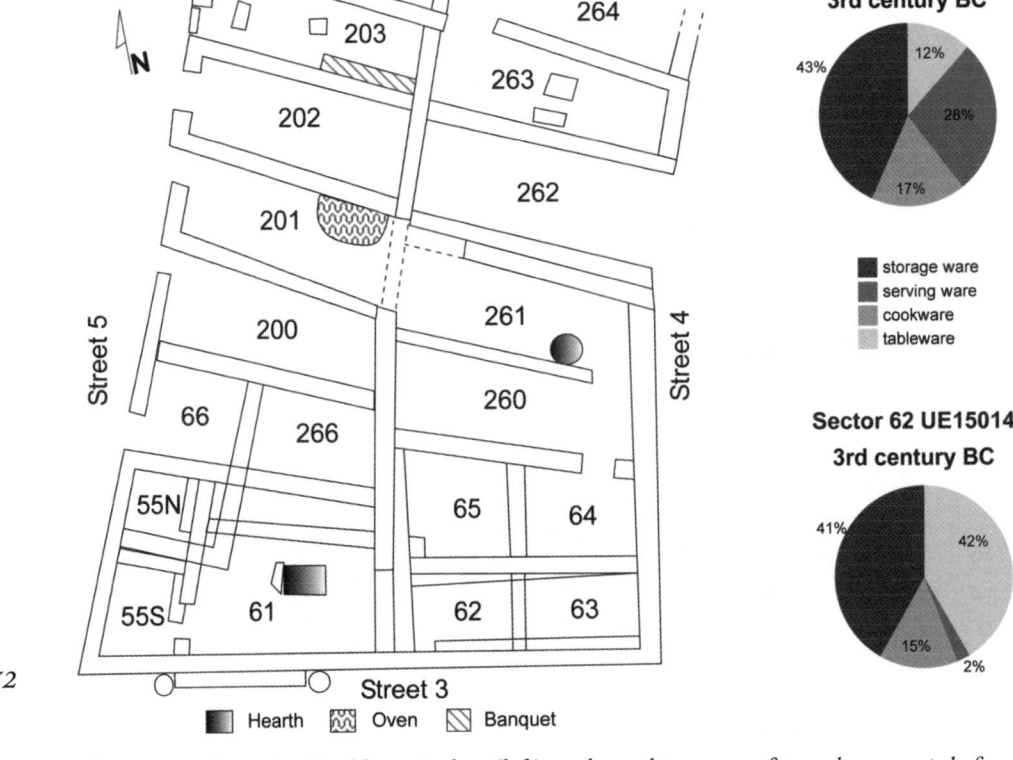

Figure 13.3. Singular Building A plan (left) and graphics quantifying the materials found (right) (M. Monrós).

These banquets differed from ordinary daily meals in the amount and the type of food and drink consumed. This indicates that food was a factor of social differentiation at that time (Pons et al. 2008, 199–200).

It is possible to characterize the organization of space in the third century BC building in relation to function. Food storage and preparation activities are found together in specialized areas within the settlement, such as Building C. In these areas we find a high percentage of storage material, together with structures for milling and hearths.

The spaces used on a daily basis for eating appear to have been located nearest the settlement walls, with the central area being occupied by more complex structures, such as Building A. The central area of this aristocratic residence may have been a meeting place in which banquets were held with the aim of legitimizing the social differences, a fact that shows us that not everybody was able to acquire imported products or large amounts of food.

References

Camañes, M.P. 2008. *Estudio estratigráfico y funcional de los espacios de molí d'espígol (tornabous, urgell): transformación, elaboración y consumo de alimentos*, inèdit.

Cura, M. 2006. *El jaciment del Molí d'Espígol (Tornabous–Urgell). Excavacions arqueològiques 1987–1992*, Barcelona, Dep. de Cultura i Mitjans de Comunicació, Monografies (Museu d'Arqueologia de Catalunya-Barcelona), 7.

Dietler, M. 1999. 'Rituals of commensality and the politics of state formation in the "princely" societies of early Iron Age Europe', *Les princes de la Protohistoire et l'émergence de l'État. Actes de la table ronde internationale de Naples (1994)*, Naples, 135–152.

Monrós, M. 2008. *La problemàtica de la reconstrucció del registre d'excavacions antigues: el cas de Molí d'Espígol (Tornabous, Urgell)*, inèdit.

Pons, E. and Garcia, L. (dir.) 2008. *Prácticas alimentarias en el mundo ibérico. El ejemplo de la fosa FS362 de Mas Castellar de Pontós (Empordà–España)*, BAR International Series, 1753.

Principal, J. 2006–2007. 'Els orígens preibèrics del Molí d'Espígol (Tornabous, l'Urgell): establiment i evolució de l'hàbitat durant la primera edat del ferro', *Revista d'Arqueologia de Ponent* 16–17, 111–128.

Principal, J., Bermúdez, X. and Saula, O. 2007. *Molí d'Espígol (Tornabous, Urgell)*. Barcelona, Museu d'Arqueologia de Catalunya.

Principal, J., Camañes, M.P. and Monrós, M. 2010. 'La ciutat ibèrica del Molí d'Espígol (Tornabous, Urgell). Darreres intervencions arqueològiques', *Urtx: Revista Cultural de l'Urgell* 24, 12–35.

Eating and Drinking with the Dead: Archaeological Evidence for Commemorative Rites at the Cemeteries of Tarraco (Tarragona, Spain) from the First to the Fourth Centuries AD

Judit Ciurana Prast
Catalan Institute of Classical Archaeology

This case study presents evidence drawn from an ongoing project aiming at analysing funerary practices and rituals at the Roman necropolis of Tarraco (Figure 14.1). This city was an outstanding Mediterranean commercial harbour and an important political and administrative centre as the capital of the *Provincia Hispania Citerior*. The *Tarraconenses* built their tombs outside the city walls and near the *via Augusta* so as to avoid a *secunda mors*, that of oblivion. Archaeology has brought two main funerary areas to light: one placed in the western suburb and another located in the eastern suburb. Even though archaeological research has directed a great deal of attention to funerary remains, ritual aspects have been comparatively neglected because of their assumed 'invisibility' within the archaeological record. Micro-stratigraphical excavation, revision of archaeological evidence and grave goods, and the study of written evidence have allowed the inferring of theories on how this funerary landscape was lived and conceived as a stage for commemorative rites.

Methodology

The aim of this project is to identify and analyse commemorative rituals performed in the funerary areas of the *suburbia* of Tarraco. In order to achieve those objectives, we have revisited museum collections and archives, and archaeological reports. The result is the study of 600 recorded burials. We have designed a complete database in FileMakerPro that gathers data related to archaeological evidence in Tarragona from the nineteenth century until the year 2008. Special fields have been created in order to collect information related to archaeological evidence on sacrifices (fauna), libations (conduits) or funerary meals (concentration of broken dishes, material installations such as fireplaces, cisterns).

Studies on religion and on the world of death in particular have been targeted towards the study of speculation about religions and gods. The major religious texts have been analysed conscientiously while ordinary ritualism has been neglected, owing to its consideration as a lower form of religion. A careful study of religious texts reveals that the essence of early Roman religion lies in the ritual practice (Scheid 2005, 8–9).

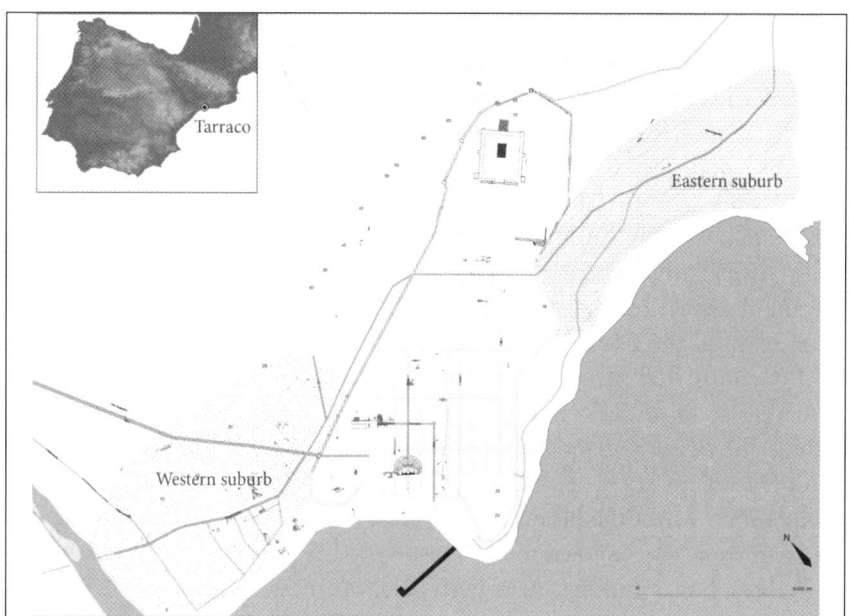

Figure 14.1. Archaeological plan of the Roman city of Tarraco. (Image provided by Planimetria Arqueològica de Tarraco (PAT 2007)).

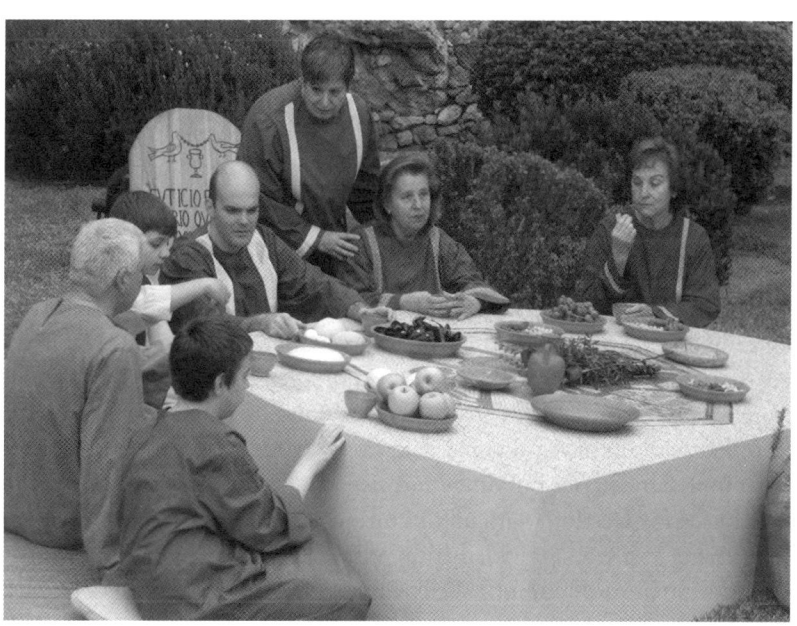

Figure 14.2: Re-enactment of a silicernium *by the Cultural Association of Saint Fructuosus (Photo: Andreu Muñoz).*

Ritual is composed of gestures and movements that leave traces in the archaeological record. These visible marks can be detected inside and outside the tombs. The funeral meal or *silicernium* was an essential part of the funerary process (Figure 14.2). Tarraco's cemeteries have revealed food offerings and eating equipment. Food found in tombs includes fruit remains (nuts, almonds), domestic animals (goat, chicken), wild animals (hare, boar) and seafood (urchins). These food offerings placed inside the tomb demonstrate that food and drink were shared with the deceased during the *funus* and marked also the sharing of a communal state of *funestas*.

Once the deceased had been cremated or his or her corpse placed in the tomb, a libation of wine to the *Manes* was poured out. This ritual practice was facilitated by the use of conduits that permitted the introduction of wine, water and milk into the grave. Libation conduits were not only used to pour liquids; the excavation of one of the conduits for *libationes* recorded in Tarraco's necropolises attested the presence of bird bones (Menchón 2000, 184). Usually these tubes are attached to one of the short sides of the tomb, where the head of the deceased was placed. There is plenty of other evidence apart from pipes and conduits attesting to the performance of libations. Cups, goblets, chalices, bowls and jugs have been discovered inside many of Tarraco's tombs. These objects were used for the reception of liquid and solid offerings that were held during sacrifices and ritual meals in the course of the funeral. The placement of jugs and cups outside the graves suggests that these drink offerings were carried out very often, especially after the funeral and during the festivals of the dead. Libation is only a part of a wider ritual but it is of significant importance because it creates a sense of order and functionality in a chaotic situation or moment. Pouring wine in honour of the deceased confirmed their status change.

Funerary landscape has to be taken into consideration because it reflects and expresses social and status structures which organize a living community. Necropolises are a cultural landscape, a 'collective representation', a sacred, symbolic replica of the living community that expressed identities, basic beliefs and values (Huntington and Metcalf 1979, 48). The material signs of the funerary areas (plots, graves and markers owned by specific families) locate these transformed dead in living time and ordered space, and so symbolically help to maintain their ongoing individual identities and affirm their continued social existence through memory. For the *Tarraconenses*, the grave was a place devoted to memory, and the act of remembrance was linked to commemorative celebrations. Excavations have provided data that demonstrate the existence of funerary gardens surrounded by service buildings and cisterns. Gardens were important, not only as a pleasant place for feasting (with all its cultural connotations), but also as a place of production. Plants and trees provided fruits, flowers and vegetables for funerary meals and for the adornment of the tomb. We have recorded two *ollae perforatae* (flowerpots) and a great number of cisterns that attest the presence of plants and trees in these gardens.

Concluding remarks

Food had a part to play in religious beliefs and practices, as is generally well-known. Eating and drinking at the tomb was also an important act of sociability, integrated into sacred space and linked to sacrifice. Offerings of food were placed at the tomb to be eaten in a funerary meal *(silicernium)* by members of the family. This study has looked at the way in which archaeology can allow us to identify ritual practices in Roman necropolises. The analysis of archaeological materials documented in the living layers of the necropolis has allowed us to detect material evidence of commemorative meals and libations. The study has also focused its attention on the evolution of these commemorative rites over the course of time. Archaeological evidence attests continuity: during four centuries, funerary meals seem to be one of those rituals that do not seem to have changed much. With the consolidation of Christianity, eating and drinking with the dead became an important cultural practice that has left ostensible signs in the archaeological record. Large concentrations of charcoal and pottery fragments related to this ritual were detected at the Early Christian necropolis of Saint Fructuosus (López Vilar 2006, 225). Funerary meals persist because they are an occasion for the remembrance of the dead and for the strengthening of social ties, something vital to overcome the trauma that death represents for the community.

References

Huntington, R. and Metcalf, P. 1979. *Celebrations of death. The anthropology of mortuary ritual*, Cambridge.
López Vilar, J. 2006. *Les basíliques paleocristianes del suburbi occidental de Tarraco*, Tarragona.
Menchón, J. 2000. 'Intervenció arqueològica al Camí de la Platja dels Cossis (Tarragona)', in Ruiz de Arbulo, J. (ed.), *Tàrraco 99. Arqueologia d'una capital provincial romana*, Tarragona, 181–189.
Scheid, J. 2005. *Quand faire, c'est croire: les rites sacrificiels des Romains*, Paris.

Relating Meat and Fish Consumption to Climate Change on the Swahili Coast (AD 700–1500)

Eréndira Quintana Morales

This paper is an introduction to current work investigating the exploitation of marine resources in coastal East Africa during a period of 800 years from 700 AD. The tropical coastlines of East Africa contain the ruins of once vibrant commercial urban settlements, where archaeologists now find long continuous records of fish consumption. Interdisciplinary methods and perspectives, borrowed from the fields of marine ecology, ethnography and archaeology, serve to reveal the interconnectedness between culture and environment in changing subsistence practices. Preliminary results in a regional analysis of faunal remains show an increasing reliance on domesticated animals, with a significant shift in the ratio of fish to domesticated animals in the twelfth century. Current research investigates this subsistence change in the context of regional climatic change.

Background

Swahili settlements are distributed along the East African coast from Somalia to Mozambique. From *c.* AD 700–1500, Swahili towns developed into essential hubs within the complex cultural network of the historical Indian Ocean trading system. Archaeologists have found, and sometimes collected, bones and shells in these settlements as evidence for subsistence strategies. However, little research has been undertaken on the changing importance of fish and shellfish consumption relative to cattle herding (for example Horton et al. 1996). Current research consolidates and contributes to Swahili subsistence data in order to understand the cultural and environmental factors associated with significant changes so far observed in fish consumption in relation to an increasing consumption of rice (Walshaw 2010) and domesticated animals.

Previous work on subsistence strategies in Africa has viewed climate as a critical pressure in the spread of domesticated plants and animals, subsistence change, and subsequently the development of complex societies. Unravelling cultural responses to climate change is complex because societies respond to environmental change according to their perception of nature and the cause of environmental change (Rosen 2007). Furthermore, different segments of society respond differently according to their perceptions and needs. Given that a society's reactions are related to their perception of the problem, which may be seen as a cultural problem or influenced by their position in society, the solution may be environmentally unsustainable but culturally reasonable. In this way the impact of the environment on humans is mediated by the responses

Relating Meat and Fish Consumption to Climate Change

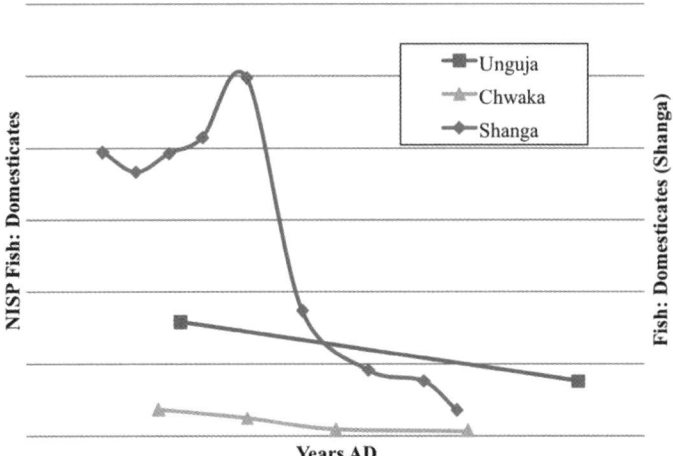

Figure 15.1. The ratio of the total number of fish bones to domesticated animal bones over time in three Swahili sites (Shanga is on the secondary axis).

of members in a society. The strategies that result from these responses influence how humans impact on their surrounding environment. Thus, this cycle of change, perception, and reaction interlinks culture and environment.

Investigating both cultural and environmental aspects provides an opportunity for marine ecologists and archaeologists to collaborate. Recent archaeological studies focusing on the history of human impact on coastal environments have incorporated methods that require knowledge of coastal ecological systems (Rick and Erlandson 2008). Additionally, ethnographies help researchers understand cultural perspectives of climate change and the social dynamics of marine resource exploitation. Currently, archaeological subsistence records from Swahili settlements are studied alongside climate data and ethnographic information. In the following paragraphs I describe the components of the interdisciplinary approach undertaken in this research.

Ichthyoarchaeology

The study of fish remains in archaeological sites provides information such as the quantity and types of fish consumed in a particular settlement over time. Records of food consumption on the East African coast are available in published faunal reports and through recently analysed excavated assemblages. The data reported here are limited to published records from three archaeological sites that contain comparable long-term chronological data: Shanga (15 ha, Horton 1996), Unguja Ukuu (16 ha, Juma 2004), and Chwaka (12–15 ha, Fleisher 2003). Although the three settlements are located at different latitude along the coast, they are all similar in size. All show a decreasing trend in the ratio of fish to domesticated animals over time (Figure 15.1). Shanga, in particular, shows a clear shift during the second half of the twelfth century. Unguja and

Relating Meat and Fish Consumption to Climate Change

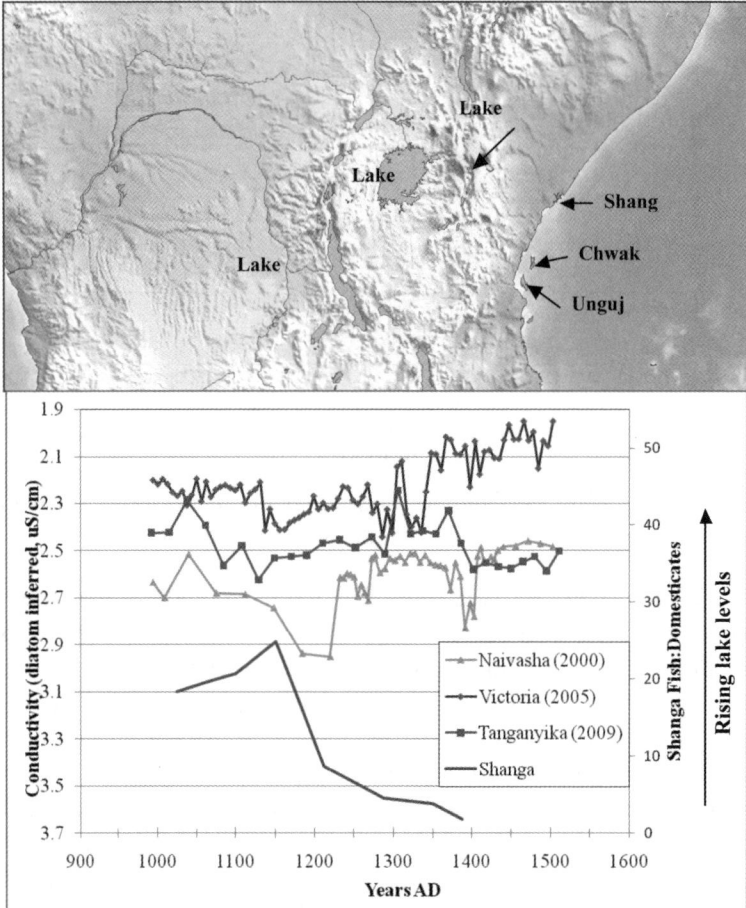

Figure 15.2: Conductivity levels through time, inferred from the diatom record, relate to lake levels. The ratio of fish to domesticated animal bones at Shanga is plotted on the secondary axis. Locations of the three archaeological studies are marked in the map.

Chwaka have more limited chronological resolution but also show a decreasing ratio of fish to domesticated animals. In order to understand the implications of this shift, the archaeological data is complemented by other forms of evidence.

Ethnoarchaeology

An ethnoarchaeology of Swahili fishing was undertaken in Vanga, Kenya and the surrounding area to understand the social dynamics and taphonomic processes of fishing and fish consumption. Fishers in Vanga area continue to use fishing methods passed down through generations in the same geographical setting as their ancestors, which allows us to make certain assumptions through continuous analogy (Stiles 1977).

Relating Meat and Fish Consumption to Climate Change

Five types of equipment represent the majority of fishing methods currently found in this area: *nyavu* (net), *lema* (basket trap), *uzio* (weir trap), *mshipi* (line), and *bunduki* (spear gun). Some of these methods are mentioned in early historical texts; for example, the use of 'baskets' for fishing is mentioned in a first century AD description of the Swahili coast in *Periplus Maris Erythraei* (Casson 1989, 59–60). Fishers in Vanga area continue to hand weave basket traps with local bark cuttings.

A collection of 60 interviews with Vanga men and women, along with observations of fishing activities, revealed that while men are mostly involved in capturing (and perhaps transporting) the marine resources, women are a crucial part of the processing and distribution within a household and a community. Generally, members of the community with higher social status consume larger quantities of domesticated animal meat than their counterparts. In the sphere of fishing, higher status is achieved by owning fishing equipment rather than participating in fishing activities. Continuing work to understand the local perceptions and dynamics of the Vanga fishing community contributes to the interpretation of the archaeological subsistence data from this area.

Paleolimnology

Environmental changes through time must also be considered in the study of subsistence change. Palaeolimnology studies of East African lakes reconstruct past climatic conditions in the region by analysing ancient sediments (Stager et al. 2009; 2005; Russell and Johnson 2007; Johnson et al. 2002; Verschuren et al. 2000). The composition of pollen, diatoms (a type of phytoplankton), and other chemical and biological traces are used as proxies for water temperature and levels. These proxies may be useful indicators of climate change in the East African region.

Overall, the East African lakes appear to be affected by a rapid decrease in lake level from the middle of the twelfth century to the first part of the thirteenth century, followed by a rapid increase in lake levels by the mid-thirteenth century (Figure 15.2). These sudden shifts, probably representing rainfall oscillation, may have had an effect on coastal environments by increasing the amount of sedimentation in the water and decreasing the amount of light, creating unfavourable conditions for a viable coral reef. Severe rainfall increases sediment runoff into the ocean. During a drought, areas of exposed soil are easily eroded into runoff with even little rain, which makes oscillating wet and dry conditions particularly likely to increase sedimentation. The effect of this phenomenon on the shifting diet of the coastal inhabitants is explored through analysis of the faunal remains.

Coral reef ecology

Fish remains data can indicate the intensity of fishing and health of an exploited marine ecological system in the past. Trophic levels indicate the feeding behaviour of marine organisms on a scale of 1 to 5, from producer (plant) to predator. While the composition of fish species may stay relatively stable through time, decreasing fish size

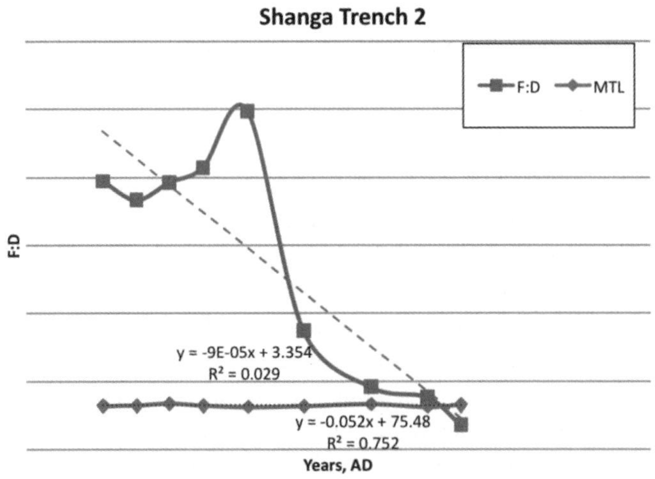

Figure 15.3. Trends in the ratio of fish bone to domesticated animal bone (F:D) and the mean trophic level (MTL) of fish bone throughout the occupation at Shanga.

and mean trophic level (MTL) of fish catch are indications of intensive fishing (Wing 2001; Pauley et al. 1998). A preliminary analysis of the MTL of fish found at Shanga shows a declining trend, representing the gradual intensification of fishing (Figure 15.3). However, there is some variation in the data, and it might be significant that one of the lowest estimates of MTL coincides with the shift from fish to domesticated animal meat. The low MTL indicates a disturbed marine system during the twelfth century.

Diet and climate interactions

A closer look at what was happening in Shanga during the twelfth century illustrates how the different interdisciplinary perspectives complement each other. Archaeological work at the site shows that at this time Shanga undergoes a phase of 'urban renewal' characterized by population growth and widespread construction (Horton 1996). The animal remains from this phase indicate a change from a diet based mainly on fish to one that includes more domesticated animal meat. Interestingly, while the ratio of fish to domesticated animal bone is quickly falling, this phase includes the highest number of fish bones. Also during this phase larger numbers of offshore pelagic fish bones begin to appear.

Historical accounts and ethnoarchaeological work have shown that domesticated animal meat is associated with ritual contexts and high social status. Could the changing diet be related to rituals associated with the ongoing construction projects, including the expansion of the Friday Mosque? More likely, the changing diet, which appears to be a regional trend, is influenced by a larger regional phenomenon related to climatic changes that may have affected the inshore marine resources and encouraged Shanga fishers to sail farther out to sea.

Conclusion

The aim of this paper was to introduce current lines of investigation in the developing field of zooarchaeology in the Swahili region. Three published long-term chronologies of faunal remains provide an outline for changing subsistence strategies on the Swahili Coast. Preliminary results show an increased reliance on domesticated faunal resources from the mid-twelfth century on a background of changing fish species composition and trophic level that indicate a disturbed marine environment; disturbed probably by humans and by a changing climate. The results also highlight the vast amount of work remaining in order to understand human-environmental relationships in this region. Current work in this field is enhanced by an interdisciplinary approach that considers the connection between humans and their environment. More detailed analysis of fish remains from Swahili sites will provide a better understanding of subsistence changes in their cultural and environmental contexts.

References

Casson, L. 1989. *The Periplus Maris Erythraei: Text with introduction, translation, and commentary*, Princeton, N.J.

Horton, M., Brown, H.W. and Mudida, N. 1996. *Shanga: The archaeology of a Muslim trading community on the coast of East Africa*, London.

Johnson, T.C., Brown, E.T., McManus, J., Barry, S.L. and Barker, P. 2002. 'A high resolution paleoclimate record spanning the past 25,000 years in southern East Africa', *Science* 296: 113–114, 131–132.

Pauley, D., Christensen, V., Dalsgaard, J., Forese, R., and Torres Jr, F. 1998. 'Fishing Down Marine Food Webs', *Science* 279(5352), 860.

Rick, T.C. and Erlandson, J. 2008. *Human impacts on ancient marine ecosystems: a global perspective*, Berkeley.

Rosen, A.M. 2007. *Civilizing climate: social responses to climate change in the ancient Near East*, Lanham.

Russell, J.M. and Johnson, T.C. 2007. 'Little Ice Age drought in equatorial Africa: Intertropical Convergence Zone migrations and El Niño–Southern Oscillation variability', *Geology* 35(1), 21–24.

Stager, J.C., Cocquyt, C., Bonnefille, C.R., Weyhenmeyer, C. and Bowerman, N. 2009. 'A late Holocene paleoclimatic history of Lake Tanganyika, East Africa', *Quaternary Research* 72, 47–56.

Stager, J.C., Ryves, D., Cumming, B.F., Meeker, L.D. and Beer, J. 2005. 'Solar variability and the levels of Lake Victoria, East Africa, during the last millennium', *Journal of Paleolimnology* 33(2), 243–251.

Stiles, D. 1977. 'Ethnoarchaeology: A Discussion of Methods and Applications', *Man* 12(1), 87–103.

Verschuren, D., Laird, K.R. and Cumming, B.F. 2000. 'Rainfall and drought in equatorial East Africa during the past 1,100 years', *Nature* 6768(403), 410–414.

Walshaw, S.C. 2010. 'Converting to rice: urbanization, Islamization and crops on Pemba Island, Tanzania, AD 700–1500', *World Archaeology* 42(1), 137–154.

Wing, E. 2001. 'The Sustainability of Resources Used by Native Americans on Four Caribbean Islands', *International Journal of Osteoarchaeology* 11, 112–126.

Reare the Goose: Recognizing a Standard Method of Carcase Dismemberment

Louisa Gidney
University of Durham

Archaeological finds

Fragments of the breast bone or sternum of geese (*Anser* sp.), sliced through parallel to the spine, had been observed by the author among faunal assemblages from medieval and post-medieval sites in north-east England, principally from Newcastle-upon-Tyne, for many years. However, the incidence of such cut marks was neither explicitly reported and the question of why the goose breast should have been cut through in this manner was not posed.

Further finds of such goose sternum fragments from medieval deposits at the New Quay, Berwick-upon-Tweed, finally prompted consideration that such fragmentation must be linked with the manner of presenting the goose meat at table (Gidney 1999, 101). For example, the illustrations in the fourteenth-century Luttrell Psalter depict geese on the spit being roasted whole (Backhouse 2000, 12) and the meat subsequently chopped up to be served at table (Backhouse 2000, 14).

A manual of carving instructions published in the seventeenth century (Murrell 1638 facs., 167–168), but repeating the description of techniques in common usage much earlier (Day 2001, 40), described a carving technique known as Reare the Goose (Appendix 1). In particular, it was thought that the phrase '*lace her downe with your knife cleane thorow the breast*' could produce the distinctive fragmentation of the goose sternum found archaeologically. Subsequent excavations at Walkergate in Berwick-upon-Tweed recovered further fragments of goose sternum sliced through the bone, from pre-sixteenth century late-medieval contexts (Archaeological Services 2007, 24), suggesting that this method of portioning goose was a commonplace practice in the town and not the preserve of higher echelons of society, as depicted in the Luttrell Psalter.

However, to date, the largest and best preserved collection of goose bones, seen by the author, showing the marks of this carving technique was recovered from sixteenth-century midden deposits in the Barbican ditch of Richmond Castle, North Yorkshire (Archaeological Services 2000). Evidence was recovered for the dismemberment of the whole goose carcase, not just the sternum. Both immature birds, with porous bones and unformed articular ends, known as green geese, and adult birds are represented in this assemblage. The contemporaneity and rapid deposition of the bones is illustrated by three pieces of one sternum that conjoin (Figures 16.1 and 16.2). A further seven pieces

Reare the Goose

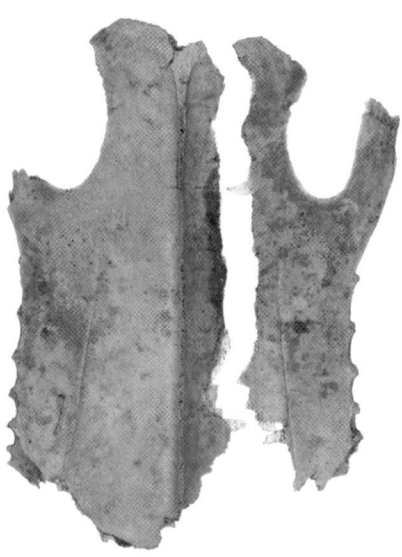

Figure 16.1. Two fragments of archaeological goose sternum from Richmond, showing the characteristic slice through the bone parallel to the spine (Photo: Jeff Veitch, Durham University).

of sternum from the same context bear witness to the method of carving discussed. Survival of this technique into the eighteenth century is indicated by a sternum fragment from a context of this period.

Modern attempts to Reare the Goose

The sliced goose bones from Richmond prompted several attempts at carving cooked geese following Murrell's instructions. These have resulted in bones that resemble the archaeological finds, as exemplified by the sterna in Figure 16.3, where the modern bones reflect the damage on the archaeological specimen in Figure 16.1. Also noteworthy are a modern coracoid and an archaeological specimen from Richmond, both of which exhibit comparable cut marks along the distal shaft. Some variation on Murrell's instructions is suggested by the archaeological pelvis fragments which, while fewer in number than those of the sternum, appear to have been cut into more, and smaller, pieces than expected from the experimental bones.

A traditional carving knife was found to be an inadequate tool to lace down the breast through the bone, so recourse was made to a robust professional cook's knife for the earlier attempts at this method. The most recent trial used a reproduction of a medieval, dagger-like, ballock knife, which worked well. Some strength, as well as skill, is needed by the carver, who also needs to be standing for the task.

Figure 16.2. View of the same goose sternum (from Richmond) showing the broken spine (Photo: Jeff Veitch, Durham University).

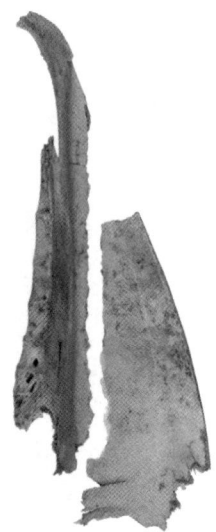

Four roast geese have been carved experimentally by Murrell's method but the spine of the sternum has not been severed on any of them, unlike the archaeological find from Richmond (Figure 16.2). However, this break may have been made by the cook rather than the carver. Thacker's eighteenth-century instructions for a goose include 'singe and flat it with a cleaver' (Day 2004, 214).

The changeover in carving style

Having ascertained how the goose bones might have been cut up, interest then focussed on how long this method of carving was in use and why and when it was superseded. By the early fifteenth century, carving was a highly formalized skill, with specific terms for the dismemberment of fish, flesh and fowl (Brears 2003). In medieval dining, the bird would have been dissected by the carver and the dish of portions presented as a mess to the diners (Brears 2003, 14). The texts (Appendices 1–2) show that the meat of the goose was carefully arranged on the serving dish, so that each diner might daintily select a piece to eat with the fingers. The bone in each portion provided a grip for the diner, comparable to a modern chicken drumstick. The description of medieval Parisian goose butchers in the fourteenth-century *Viandier* of Taillevent (Scully 1988, 283) may suggest that medieval town-dwellers could have their cooked bird cut up by a professional carver before consumption at home, leading to the standardized fragments of goose sterna seen in the archaeological record from Berwick and Richmond. The French roast geese were 'cut up into pieces and slices in such a way that in each piece there is skin, flesh and bone; and they do it very neatly' (Scully 1988, 283), which suggests that the French method of carving was broadly comparable to the Reare the Goose style. This style of portioning was designed to facilitate dainty eating with fingers.

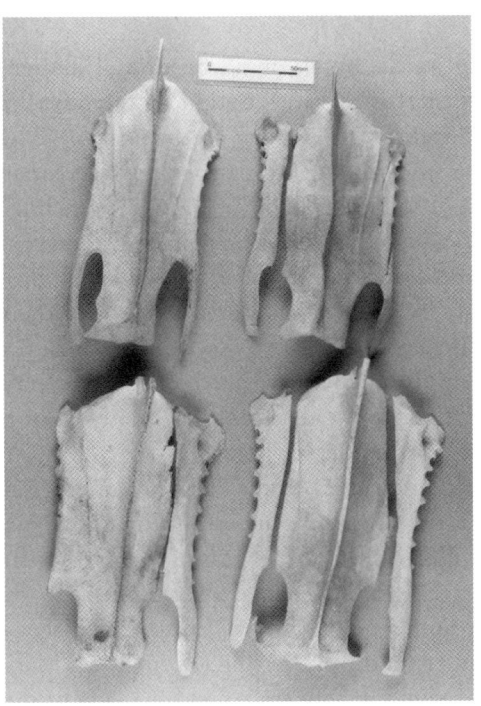

Figure 16.3. Modern goose sterna. Three carved by the reare the goose method and one by the modern method (Photo: Jennifer Jones, Durham University).

From the sixteenth century, printed books made this information on carving and dining etiquette available to a broad clientele, desirous of emulating the manners of the landed gentry (Brears 2003, 3). Murrell's 1638 directions (Appendix 1) to Reare a Goose were already at least two centuries old but continued as standard practice and terminology into the mid-eighteenth century, for example the directions to rear a goose in the 1758 edition of Eliza Smith (Appendix 2) still follow those of Murrell closely. The connection of such cookery writers with noble households is generally strongly promoted as a selling point. Eliza Smith (1758 facs., A4), for example, emphasized her 30 years employment by fashionable and noble families and that her recipes were practical for frugal, genteel and noble tables.

By the 1791 edition of Trusler's *Honours of the Table* (Appendix 3), the influence of the old style of carving remains evident but change is indicated. Trusler uses new phraseology, tied to an illustration which is essential to understand the instructions. The breast is still carved in slices downwards, but only to the bone, not through it. Explicit reference is also made to the use of a fork in manipulating the goose to remove the legs. Trusler observes that the same method of carving applies to a green goose as to an old bird, as seen for the earlier archaeological specimens from Richmond.

During the earlier nineteenth century, the old style of carving was superseded by the modern style of cutting slices upwards from the wing to the spine of the breast, removing the meat from the bone. The new carving style was publicized by all subsequent cookery authors, most famously Mrs Beeton in 1861 (Appendix 4).

Forks for carving and dining

The demise of the old style of carving on the buffet or sideboard and dining from a communal mess with the fingers coincides with the adoption of the table fork and individual place settings in the later eighteenth century (Brown 2001). By 1810, a schoolboy was taught to lay down the silver dining fork and use a steel carving fork when helping the adjacent ladies to a portion of game bird (Anon 1810, 231).

The carving forks that were slowly adopted by the gentry during the seventeenth century have short tines to hold the meat steady (Day 2001, 33), replacing the fingers or a second knife, while the carving knife sliced downwards, away from the carver's fork hand, as in the example under discussion to Reare a Goose. This style of carving generally required the carver to stand and was the prerogative of the gentleman. The carving fork with finger guard is the indispensable adjunct for the more recent method of carving slices upwards from the goose breast, off the bone.

Carving forks were not manufactured in quantity by the Sheffield cutlery trade prior to the nineteenth century (Symonds 2002). The introduction of the finger guard and the widespread adoption of the carving fork reflect the increasing changeover from the old to new style of carving, mirroring the gradual change from dining *à la française*, with many dishes served on the table simultaneously, to *à la russe* with a sequence of individual courses and the requisite cutlery and place setting (Brears 1994; Mars 1994). With the new carving forks, the carver could remain seated and the lady of the house could share the task (Mars 1994, 138–9). Mrs Beeton (Appendix 4) was describing the ongoing take-up of the new style of carving, using an implement that had relatively recently become a commonplace artefact of the burgeoning, aspirational, middle classes. The roast bird remained the focus of household table ceremonial but the style of portioning changed with the introduction of individual plates of food eaten with knife and fork replacing the communal mess eaten with the fingers.

Conclusion

The finds from medieval towns of archaeological goose bones showing evidence of portioning by the Reare the Goose method demonstrate that this technique was commonplace and not a table etiquette confined by social class. The dissemination of printed instructions for carving from the sixteenth century onwards may be reflected in standardization in the method of cutting up the cooked goose and so in the archaeological finds of goose bones. The perusal of eighteenth-century cookery texts demonstrates that the eighteenth-century deposit from Richmond containing goose bones cut up by the Reare the Goose method is not an anachronistic find.

The change to dining with knife and fork from a plate and concomitant development of the carving fork for slicing the breast meat of the goose upwards towards the spine rather than downwards onto, or through, the breast bone is very recent. Only a well stratified sequence of eighteenth- to nineteenth-century deposits would chronicle this changeover archaeologically.

Reare the Goose

The matching carving knife and fork sets of the nineteenth century onwards were designed for slicing neatly through meat, not bone, hence the problems encountered when endeavouring to Reare a Goose with such a blade.

References

Anon. 1810. *Letters from a Nobleman to His Son*, 1, London.
Archaeological Services. 2000. *The Barbican of Richmond Castle, North Yorkshire*, Archaeological Services Durham University Report 663.
Archaeological Services. 2007. *Berwick-upon-Tweed Walkergate Workspace Project, Northumberland: plant macrofossil, faunal remains, vessel and industrial residue analysis*, Archaeological Services Durham University Report 1780.
Backhouse, J. 2000. *Medieval Rural Life in the Luttrell Psalter*, London.
Beeton, I. 1861. Facs. ed. 1982. *Book of Household Management*, London.
Brears, P. 1994. 'A la Française: the Waning of a Long Dining Tradition', in Wilson, C.A. (ed.), *Luncheon, Nuncheon and Other Meals*, Stroud, 91–116.
Brears, P. (ed.) 2003. *The Book of Keruynge*, Lewes.
Brown, P. (ed.) 2001. *British Cutlery. An Illustrated History of Design, Evolution and Use*, London.
Day, I. 2001. 'The Honours of the Table', in Brown, P. (ed.), *British Cutlery. An Illustrated History of Design, Evolution and Use*, London, 32–42.
Day, I. (ed.) 2004. *The Art of Cookery by John Thacker, 1758*, Lewes.
Gidney, L.J. 1999. 'The animal bones', in Griffiths, W.B. (ed.), Excavations at the New Quay, Berwick-upon-Tweed, 1996, *Archaeologia Aeliana 5th Series* XXVII, 100–102
Mars, V. 1994. 'A la Russe: The New Way of Dining', in Wilson C.A. (ed.), *Luncheon, Nuncheon and Other Meals*, Stroud, 117–144.
Murrell, J. 1638. Facs, ed.1985. *Two Books of Cookery and Carving*, Ilkley.
Scully, T. 1988. *The Viandier of Taillevent*, Ottawa.
Smith, E. 1758. Facs. ed. 1994. *The Compleat Housewife*, London.
Symonds, J. (ed.) 2002. *The Historical Archaeology of the Sheffield Cutlery and Tableware Industry 1750–1900*, BAR Brit. Ser. 341, Oxford.
Trusler, J. 1791. *The Honours of the Table*, Dublin.

Appendix: Published directions for carving goose
1. Reare the Goose (Murrell 1638. Facs. ed. 1985, 167–8)
You must breake a Goose up contrary to this fashion. Take a Goose being roasted, and take of both the Legges faire like a shoulder of Lambe, take them quite from the body, then cut off the belly piece round, close to the lower end of the brest: then lace her downe with your knife cleane thorow the breast, on each side your Thumbs breadth from the bone in the middle of the breast. Then take off the Pinion of each side, and the flesh which you first laced with your knife, raise it up cleane from the bone, and take it cleane from the carkasse with the Pinion. Then cut up the bone which lyeth before in the breast, which you commonly call the Merry thought, the skin and the flesh being upon it. Then cut from the breast bone another slice of flesh cleane thorow, and take it cleane from the bone

: then turne your carkasse, and cut it asunder, the backe bone above the loyne bones, then take the Rumpe end of the Back-bone, and lay it in a faire Dish, with the skinne side upward, lay at the fore-end of it the Merry-thought, with the skinne side upward, and before that the apron of the Goose : then lay your Pinions on each side contrary, set your legges on each side contrary behinde them, that the bone end of the legges may stand up crosse in the middle of the Dish, and the Wing Pinions may come on the outside of them. Put under the Wing Pinions on each side the long slices of flesh which you cut from the breast bone, and let the ends meet under the legge-bones, and let the other ends lie cut in the Dish betwixt the Leg and the Pinion: then powre in your sauce into the Dish under your meate, then throw on Salt, and set it on the Table.

2. To rear a Goose (Smith 1758. Facs. ed 1994, 393)
Take off both legs fair, like shoulders of lamb; then cut off the belly-piece round close to the end of the breasr; then lace your goose down on both sides of the breast half an inch from the sharp bone; then take off the pinion on each side, and the flesh you first lac'd with your knife; raise it clean from the bone, and take it off with the pinion from the body; then cut up the merry-thought; then cut from the breast bone another slice of flesh quite thro'; then turn up your carcase, and cut it asunder, the back-bone above the loin-bones; then take the rump end of the back-bone and lay it in a dish, with the skinny side up-wards; lay at the fore-end of it the merry-thought, with the skinny-side upwards, and before that the apron of the goose; then lay the pinions on each side contrary, set the legs on each side contrary behind them, that the bone ends of the legs may stand up cross in the middle of the dish, and the wing pinions may come on the outside of them; put the long slice which you cut from the breast-bone, under the wing pinions on each side, and let the ends meet under the leg bones, and let the other ends lie cut in the dish betwixt the leg and the pinion; then pour in your sauce under the meat; throw on salt, and serve it to table again.

3. A Goose (Trusler 1791, 53–56)
Like a turkey, is seldom quite dissected, unless the company is large; but when it is, the following is the method. Turn the neck towards you, and cut two or three long slices, on each side of the breast, in the lines *a b*, quite to the bone. Cut these slices from the bone, which done, proceed to take off the leg, by turning the goose up on one side putting the fork through the small end of the leg-bone, pressing it close to the body, which when the knife is entered at *d* raises the joint from the body. The knife is then to be passed under the leg in the direction *d e*. If the leg hangs to the carcase at the joint *e*, turn it back with the fork, and it will readily separate, if the goose is young: in an old goose it will require some strength to separate it. When the leg is off, proceed to take off the wing, by

passing the fork through the small end of the pinion, pressing it close to the body and entering the knife at the notch *c* and passing it under the wing in the direction *c d*. It is a nice thing to hit this notch *c*, as it is not so visible in the bird as in the figure. If the knife is put into the notch above it, you cut upon the neck bone and not on the wing joint. A little practice will soon teach the difference, and if the goose is young, the trouble is not great, but very much otherwise, if the bird is an old one.

When the leg and wing on one side are taken off, take them off on the other side; cut off the apron in the line *f e g*, and then take off the merry-thought in the line *i h*. The neck-bones are next to be separated as in a fowl, and all other parts divided as there directed, to which I refer you.

The best parts of a goose are in the following order; the breast slices; the fleshy part of the wing, which may be divided from the pinion; the thigh bone, which may be easily divided in the joint from the leg-bone, or drum-stick, as it is called, the pinion and next the side-bones. To those who like sage and onion, draw it out with a spoon from the body, at the place where the apron is taken from, and mix it with the gravy, which should first be poured from the boat into the body of the goose, before anyone is helped. The rump is a nice bit to those who like it. It is often peppered and salted, and sent down to be boiled, and is then called a Devil, as I have mentioned in speaking of a turkey. Even the carcase of a goose, by some, is preferred to other parts, as being more juicy and more savory.

A Green Goose is cut up the same way, but the most delicate part is the breast and the gristle, at the lower part of it.

4. Roast Goose (Beeton 1861. Facs. ed. 1982, 501; 504–5)

A tough fowl and an old goose are sad triers of a carver's powers and temper, and, indeed, sometimes of the good humour of those in the neighbourhood of the carver.

It would not be fair to say that this dish bodes a great deal of happiness to an inexperienced carver, especially if there is a large party to serve, and the slices off the breast should not suffice to satisfy the desires and cravings of many wholesome appetites…..

The beginning of the task, however is not in any way difficult. Evenly-cut slices, not too thick or too thin, should be carved from the breast in the direction of the line from 2 to 3; after the first slice has been cut, a hole should be made with the knife in the part called the apron, passing it round the line, as indicated by the figures 1, 1, 1,: here the stuffing is located…..

If the carver manages cleverly, he will be able to cut a very large number of fine slices off the breast, and the more so if he commences close down by the wing, and carves upwards towards the ridge of the breastbone…….